MEALS IN SCHOOL: ISSUES AND IMPACTS

FOOD AND BEVERAGE CONSUMPTION AND HEALTH

Additional books in this series can be found on Nova's website under the Series tab.

Additional E-books in this series can be found on Nova's website under the E-books tab.

FOOD AND BEVERAGE CONSUMPTION AND HEALTH

MEALS IN SCHOOL: ISSUES AND IMPACTS

DAYNA A. MICHALKA
AND
CHRISTOPHER J. MONROY
EDITORS

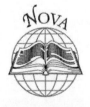

Nova Science Publishers, Inc.
New York

Copyright © 2011 by Nova Science Publishers, Inc.

NOTICE TO THE READER

The Publisher has taken reasonable care in the preparation of this book, but makes no expressed or implied warranty of any kind and assumes no responsibility for any errors or omissions. No liability is assumed for incidental or consequential damages in connection with or arising out of information contained in this book. The Publisher shall not be liable for any special, consequential, or exemplary damages resulting, in whole or in part, from the readers' use of, or reliance upon, this material. Any parts of this book based on government reports are so indicated and copyright is claimed for those parts to the extent applicable to compilations of such works.

Independent verification should be sought for any data, advice or recommendations contained in this book. In addition, no responsibility is assumed by the publisher for any injury and/or damage to persons or property arising from any methods, products, instructions, ideas or otherwise contained in this publication.

This publication is designed to provide accurate and authoritative information with regard to the subject matter covered herein. It is sold with the clear understanding that the Publisher is not engaged in rendering legal or any other professional services. If legal or any other expert assistance is required, the services of a competent person should be sought. FROM A DECLARATION OF PARTICIPANTS JOINTLY ADOPTED BY A COMMITTEE OF THE AMERICAN BAR ASSOCIATION AND A COMMITTEE OF PUBLISHERS.

Additional color graphics may be available in the e-book version of this book.

LIBRARY OF CONGRESS CATALOGING-IN-PUBLICATION DATA

Meals in school : issues and impacts / Dayna A. Michalka and Christopher J. Monroy [editors].
p. cm. -- (Food and beverage consumption and health)
Includes bibliographical references and index.
ISBN 978-1-61209-127-3 (hardcover : alk. paper)
1. School children--Food. 2. Children--Nutrition. 3. School breakfast programs. I. Michalka, Dayna A. II. Monroy, Christopher J.
LB3473.M43 2011
371.7'16--dc22
2010047020

Published by Nova Science Publishers, Inc. † New York

CONTENTS

PREFACE

Participation in the School Breakfast Program is much less common than participation in the National School Lunch Program, even among children with access to both programs. Studies have found that students are more likely to participate when breakfast is served in the classroom, when time available for breakfast in school is longer, and when they come from lower income or time-constrained households. This new book examines the determinants of participation in the School Breakfast Program, as well as the impacts of the program on food insecurity and children's risk of skipping breakfast.

Chapter 1- The School Breakfast Program is an important component of the nutritional safety net, serving over 10 million children per day. Despite the scope of the program, it is less widely available and less consistently used than the National School Lunch Program. There remains substantial variability, both across and within states, in the extent to which it is available and the degree to which students participate, and the factors related to this variability are not well understood. And, while some benefits of the program have been well documented, the impact of the program on other outcomes, including food insecurity and breakfast-skipping, remains unclear.

Chapter 2- The School Breakfast Program is a federally assisted meal program operating in public and nonprofit private schools and residential child care institutions. It began as a pilot project in 1966, and was made permanent in 1975. The School Breakfast Program is administered at the Federal level by the Food and Nutrition Service. At the State level, the program is usually administered by State education agencies, which operate the program through agreements with local school food authorities in more than 87,000 schools and institutions.

Chapter 3- Concerns about child obesity have raised questions about the quality of meals served in the National School Lunch Program. Local, State, and Federal policymakers responded to these concerns beginning in the mid-1990s by instituting a range of policies and standards to improve the quality of U.S. Department of Agriculture-subsidized meals. Schools have been successful in meeting USDA nutrient standards except those for total fat and saturated fat. This chapter uses school-level data from the School Nutrition Dietary Assessment-III to calculate statistical differences between the fat content of NSLP lunches served by schools with different policies (e.g., menu planning) and characteristics like region and size. Positive associations are found between a meal's fat content and the presence of a la carte foods and vending machines, which are thought to indirectly affect the nutrient content of USDA-subsidized meals.

Chapter 4- Changing small factors that influence consumer choice may lead to healthier eating within controlled settings, such as school cafeterias. This chapter describes a behavioral experiment in a college cafeteria to assess the effects of various payment options and menu selection methods on food choices. The results indicate that payment options, such as cash or debit cards, can significantly affect food choices. College students using a card that prepaid only for healthful foods made more nutritious choices than students using either cash or general debit cards. How and when individuals select their food can also influence food choices. College students who preselected their meals from a menu board made significantly different food choices than students who ordered their meals while viewing the foods in line.

In: Meals in School: Issues and Impacts   ISBN: 978-1-61209-127-3
Editors: Dayna A. Michalka et al.   © 2011 Nova Science Publishers, Inc.

Chapter 1

THE SCHOOL BREAKFAST PROGRAM

Judi Bartfeld, Myoung Kim, Jeong Hee Ryu,
and Hong-Min Ahn

ABSTRACT

Participation in the School Breakfast Program is much less common than participation in the National School Lunch Program, even among children with access to both programs. This chapter examines the determinants of participation in the School Breakfast Program among third grade public school students, as well as the impacts of the program on food insecurity and children's risk of skipping breakfast. Data are from the Early Childhood Longitudinal Survey— Kindergarten Cohort and from the Wisconsin Schools Food Security Survey. The study found that students are more likely to participate when breakfast is served in the classroom, when time available for breakfast in school is longer, and when they come from lower income or time-constrained households. Children with access to the School Breakfast Program are more likely to eat breakfast in the morning and that program access may enhance food security among families at the margin of food insecurity.

EXECUTIVE SUMMARY

The School Breakfast Program is an important component of the nutritional safety net, serving over 10 million children per day. Despite the scope of the program, it is less widely available and less consistently used than the National School Lunch Program. There remains substantial variability, both across and within states, in the extent to which it is available and the degree to which students participate, and the factors related to this variability are not well understood. And, while some benefits of the program have been well documented, the impact of the program on other outcomes, including food insecurity and breakfast-skipping, remains unclear.

What is the Issue?

This chapter is intended to shed light both on the determinants of participation in the School Breakfast Program, and on some of the potential benefits of the program on children, using more recent data than has been available in most existing analyses. First, we focus on patterns and predictors of participation in the School Breakfast Program among third-grade students in public schools nationwide, contrasting participation patterns in school breakfast with those in school lunch, where the latter is much more widely available and utilized. Next, we explore the impact of the School Breakfast Program on food insecurity, focusing on differences between low- income children who do and do not have access to the program at their school. Finally, we examine the impact of the School Breakfast Program on the likelihood that children skip breakfast.

What Did the Study Find?

Our analysis confirms that school breakfast is much less widely used than school lunch, even among children with access to both programs. Furthermore, breakfast participation is almost entirely limited to a subset of the students who regularly eat school lunch. The program appears to serve as an expanded way of utilizing school meals for a subset of the students already predisposed to such meals; it receives only extremely limited use among other students. And, more so than school lunch, school breakfast appears to be used primarily by the subset of students who are most vulnerable. At the same time, there remains a substantial share of at-risk children who have access to the program yet do not participate—including 38 percent of those who are food insecure.

Multivariate analyses suggest that both economic vulnerability and time constraints are linked to participation, with low income and education, more children, and having two employed parents in the home emerging as significant predictors. We also find indirect evidence that local norms may be important in the participation decision, as evidenced by significantly higher participation in schools with a larger share of low-income students, as well as in neighborhoods with lower median incomes. Furthermore, it appears the normative nature of participation in low-income schools may have spillover effects on higher income children who might otherwise be less inclined to participate. Pronounced differences in participation according to race and ethnicity could also reflect differences in norms or preferences. On the other hand, and counter to our expectation, we found less likelihood of participation among children living in counties with more liberal political climates, suggesting that prevailing wisdom about political norms and attitudes towards public programs may not be reflected in school meal program decisions.

Of particular interest, we found that programmatic and logistical aspects of how breakfast is structured at the school are significantly linked to the likelihood of participation. Results strongly support the hypothesis that increasing the convenience of the School Breakfast Program leads to greater participation, with evidence of the importance of where breakfast is offered (classroom versus cafeteria), the duration of the breakfast period, and the arrival time of buses relative to the start of classes. While smaller-scale local studies have found evidence that features such as in-class breakfast increase participation, this is the first evidence, to our knowledge, of its impact on a national scale.

Our findings suggest that school breakfast availability is linked to a lower probability of marginal food security among low-income children, though not to food insecurity at the standard threshold. That is, the program appears beneficial in offsetting food-related concerns among at- risk families, though not necessarily in alleviating food insecurity once hardships have crossed the food insecurity threshold. While it is possible that unmeasured differences between schools that do and do not offer the program could bias our results, we find it more plausible that any bias would result in underestimates, rather than overestimates, of the true impact, given that school breakfast is disproportionately offered in schools with higher-need populations, at least based on observable characteristics. On the other hand, we were unable to substantiate our findings with an instrumental variable model, despite the existence of a strong state policy instrument. We note the relatively small number of low-income students in our sample who do not have access to school breakfast, thus hampering our ability to obtain more precise estimates of program impact.

We also found that availability of the School Breakfast Program significantly reduces the probability of skipping at least one breakfast per week, and in particular, that offering breakfast at school serves to moderate the risk of breakfast-skipping associated with low income.

Taken as a whole, our findings indicate that access to the School Breakfast Program yields significant benefits in terms of enhancing food security among families at the margin of food insecurity, and increasing the probability that children—particularly low-income children—eat breakfast in the morning. Our findings suggest that making school breakfast more broadly available would be beneficial in ensuring that more children start their school day with a meal, and that fewer families are confronted with uncertain access to sufficient food. Furthermore, our findings on participation patterns suggest that these benefits could also be enhanced with greater participation among children who already have access to the program.

How Was the Study Conducted?

We used the third-grade wave of the Early Childhood Longitudinal Survey Kindergarten Cohort (ECLS-K) to estimate probit models of students' participation in SBP, as well as probit and instrumental variable models of food security of students' households. The ECLS-K is a national survey providing data on, among other things, the availability of and participation in school meal programs as well as food security status and a range of other child outcomes. In addition, we used data from the Wisconsin Schools Food Security Survey to estimate probit and instrumental variable models of breakfast-skipping.

THE SCHOOL BREAKFAST PROGRAM: PARTICIPATION AND IMPACTS

The School Breakfast Program is an important component of the nutritional safety net, serving over 10 million children per day (Food Research and Action Center 2007). Despite the scope of the program, it is less widely available and less consistently used than the National School Lunch Program. There remains substantial variability, both across and within states, in the extent to which it is available and the degree to which students participate, and the factors related to this variability are not well understood. Furthermore, the impact of the program on various measures of child wellbeing remains uncertain, due in part to hard-to-measure differences between localities that do and don't offer the program and between students who do and don't choose to participate (see, e.g., Fox, Hamilton, and Lin 2004).

This chapter is intended to shed light both on the determinants of participation in the School Breakfast Program, and on some of the potential benefits of the program on children, using more recent data than has been available in most existing analyses. First, we focus on patterns and predictors of participation in the School Breakfast Program among third-grade students in public schools nationwide, contrasting participation patterns in school breakfast with those in school lunch, where the latter is much more widely available and utilized. We use data from the Early Childhood Longitudinal Survey – Kindergarten Cohort (ECLS-K), third grade wave, a national survey providing data on, among other things, the availability of and participation in school meal programs as well as food security status and a range of other child outcomes. Next, we use the ECLS-K data to explore the impact of the School Breakfast Program on food insecurity, focusing on differences between low income children who do and do not have access to the program at their school. Finally, we examine the impact of the School Breakfast Program on the likelihood that children skip breakfast, using data from a self- administered survey of parents of elementary school children in Wisconsin, collected during 2003-2005.

BACKGROUND

The School Breakfast Program is an important part of the nutritional safety net. Funded by the federal government and administered locally by schools and school districts around the country, the program offers all children in participating schools an opportunity to eat a low-cost, or sometimes free, breakfast either prior to or during the school day. The School Breakfast Program operates in more than 85,000 public and nonprofit private schools and residential child care institutions. School districts and independent schools that choose to take part in the program receive cash subsidies from the U.S. Department of Agriculture (USDA) for each meal they serve, and agree to serve breakfasts that meet federal program requirements. Children whose families have income below 130 percent of the federal poverty line receive free meals; children whose family incomes are between 130 percent and 185 percent of the poverty line receive reduced-price meals (costing no more than 30 cents); and children above this threshold pay full price. Schools are provided some federal reimbursement for all participating children, with higher reimbursement rates for children who are eligible for free or reduced price meals (U.S. Department of Agriculture 2008).

Participation in School Breakfast Program

Despite considerable evidence that eating breakfast has beneficial impacts on children (see Gleason and Suitor 2001, p1 8-19, for overview), availability of and participation in the School Breakfast Program continue to trail comparable indicators for the National School Lunch Program. Nationwide, approximately 85 percent of schools that offer school lunch also offer breakfast (Food Research and Action Center 2007), although this varies considerably among states – from a low of 52 percent to a high of 100 percent. When breakfast is available at school, past research suggests that only 18 percent of children participate on a given day, as compared to 62 percent participating in school lunch (Gordon and Fox 2007). And, past research has shown that participation is heavily tilted towards students who receive subsidized meals: students approved for free meals have participation rates of 39 percent, as compared to 20 percent for students approved for reduced-price meals and 8 percent among students who pay full price (Fox et al 2001). In fiscal year 2008, 80.6 percent of school breakfasts served were to students who received free or reduced price meals (Food and Nutrition Service).

The most recent information on characteristics of participants and nonparticipants, as well as determinants of participation, is from the School Nutrition and Dietary Assessment Survey-III (SNDA-III). Both descriptive and multivariate analyses suggest that, among students with access to the program, participation is more common among boys than girls, among elementary school children as compared to older children, and among nonwhite children as compared to white children. Students who are income eligible for free or reduced price meals are more likely to participate than are higher income students, and students in rural areas are more likely to participate than are their urban counterparts (Gordon et al 2007). Other research on School Breakfast Program participation examines perceived barriers rather than formal predictors of participation. Common themes from that body of research include stigma associated with the program, time conflicts associated with eating school breakfast prior to the start of the school day, and a belief that parents should be responsible for feeding their own children in the morning (see, e.g. Kennedy and Davis 1998; Lent and Emerson 2007; Reddan, Wahlstrom, and Reicks 2002; Rosales and Janowski 2002). This work suggests that both community norms as well as details of how the program is implemented that could reduce stigma and time conflicts should have beneficial impacts on participation. Initial research is consistent with this expectation: Making school breakfast available at no cost (i.e. universal free breakfast) is strongly linked to higher participation rates, based on comparisons of schools with and without a universal program (Bernstein et al 2004; Lent and Emerson 2006). There is also suggestive evidence that universal breakfast is particularly beneficial to participation when breakfast is offered during the classroom as part of the school day rather than before school (Bernstein et al 2004; Wong and Emerson 2006), although this has not received careful research attention. Among students in the SNDA-III who did not usually eat school breakfast, more than half indicated they would be more likely to do so if it were served in the classroom (Gordon et al 2007).

Almost entirely absent from the literature on School Breakfast Program participation is any formal attention to the role of the local programmatic, economic or social/political climate. This absence is striking, considering the well documented impact of such factors on caseloads in other assistance programs (see, e.g., Figlio, Gundersen, and Ziliak 2000; Ziliak, Gundersen, and Figlio 2003 for examples of studies linking macroeconomic and political indicators to food stamp caseloads). Certainly perceptions about the role of stigma and community norms are consistent with a role for contextual factors in influencing participation. With regard to programmatic characteristics, Gordon et al (2007) do find evidence that the cost of school breakfast is linked to the likelihood of participation, with higher costs associated with lower participation. On the other hand, they found no evidence of a role for several other program attributes including the form of delivery (offer versus serve);

the type of menu planning system (food-based versus nutrient standard); the percent of calories from fat; or whether meals were prepared onsite.

This chapter explores School Breakfast Program participation among third-grade public school students in a national sample. We use recent data to examine participation patterns among a very specific age group, rather than looking collectively at multiple age groups that might have varying determinants of participation. We pay particular attention to the role of operational features of the program as well as contextual characteristics intended to proxy for local norms and economic conditions.

Impacts of School Breakfast Program on Selected Outcomes

The School Breakfast Program could potentially have a range of impacts on children and families. By offering a source of breakfast—school-based meals—that would not otherwise be available, it could alter eating patterns, affecting the likelihood of eating breakfast, the location of breakfast (home versus school), and/or the kinds of food eaten. Likewise, by providing children with access to subsidized breakfasts—for some children free or at very low cost—it could reduce the risk of food-related hardships. By altering eating patterns, it could, ultimately, affect affect nutritional, health, cognitive, and other kinds of outcomes. We provide a brief overview of what is currently known about the impacts of the School Breakfast Program on two outcomes that are the focus of this chapter—food insecurity and breakfast skipping. For a detailed discussion of the impact of the School Breakfast Program on other outcomes, see Fox, Hamilton and Lin (2004).

Impacts of School Breakfast Program on Food Insecurity

Efforts to identify the impact of food assistance programs on food insecurity are complicated by self-selection into programs on the basis of unobservable characteristics, with persons at greater risk of food insecurity more likely to participate. Indeed, bivariate statistics and many multivariate analyses typically reveal the counterintuitive finding that participants in food assistance programs have higher rates of food insecurity than do nonparticipants, even when limited to the low income, suggesting important underlying differences in risk of food insecurity between participants and nonparticipants (see, e.g., Wilde 2007, for discussion of the literature on food stamps and food insecurity).

Looking across food assistance programs, analyses that do not rely solely on individual measures of program participation have found some evidence of beneficial impacts on food security. For instance, Bartfeld and Dunifon (2006) found that near-poor households in states with higher food stamp participation rates have lower risk of food insecurity, and Bernell, Weber and Edwards (2004) found that higher county-level food stamp participation is linked to reduced risk of food insecurity among households in Oregon. Yen and colleagues (2007) documented a negative impact of food stamp participation on food insecurity, using an instrumental variable approach utilizing state policy differences including the length of the food stamp recertification period. Likewise, Bartfeld and Dunifon (2006) found that households in states with higher participation in summer food programs have lower risk of food insecurity, and Nord and Romig (2006) found that seasonal differences in food insecurity (higher in the summer than the spring) are smaller in states with more widespread participation in the Summer Food Service program, providing suggestive evidence that the program helps ameliorate food insecurity among households with school-aged children.

Research on the relationship between the School Breakfast Program and food security lags behind such research on other food assistance programs. To date, no research has documented a link between the School Breakfast Program and household food security. Bartfeld and Dunifon (2006) found no significant relationship between the state participation rate of low- income children in the School Breakfast Program (benchmarked against participation of low- income children in the School Lunch Program) and food security, and likewise, Bartfeld and Wang (2006) found no evidence that the estimated participation rate among eligible children is linked to food insecurity, using data from Wisconsin. Comparing students in schools with universal-free school breakfast to a control group without universal-free breakfast, McLaughlin et al (2002) found no difference in the likelihood of food insecurity.

Because the School Breakfast Program is only available in a subset of schools, it is possible to look at program availability, and not merely program participation, to assess impacts on food insecurity. Research to date has not addressed this question. There are reasons, though, to hypothesize that access to the School Breakfast Program could reduce food insecurity. Participation is highly concentrated among the low income, where the greatest food insecurity risk is found, and among participating children, school breakfast is linked to clear changes in nutrition outcomes (see, e.g., Fox, Hamilton, and Lin 2004). Furthermore, Bhattacharya, Currie and Haider (2004) found some evidence that availability of the School Breakfast Program contributes to improved diet quality even among other family members, suggesting that participation affects broader patterns of food consumption in the household. In this chapter, we examine the relationship between the School Breakfast Program and food insecurity, using a national sample of third grade public school students. Our primary strategy is to compare household food insecurity among students with and without access to the program, controlling for observable attributes of students, households, and communities; we explore the use of instrumental variable models to further control for unmeasured differences in program availability.

Impacts of School Breakfast Program on Breakfast-Skipping

An important stream of research has considered whether the School Breakfast Program increases the likelihood that students eat breakfast on school days (or equivalently, whether it decreases the likelihood of skipping breakfast). Despite the importance of this question to policymakers interested in gauging the impacts of the program, the evidence here is mixed. The continuing uncertainly appears to be due in part to variation in how breakfast is defined, and in part to difficulty in documenting program impacts in the absence of random assignment—a pervasive concern in the broader literature on impacts of nutrition assistance programs.

Initial research from the School Nutrition Dietary Assessment Study (SNDA) found no evidence that the availability of the School Breakfast Program is linked to greater likelihood of eating breakfast (Gleason 1995). However, a reanalysis of the SNDA using more rigorous definitions of breakfast and looking separately at impacts for children at different income levels found that, when a more stringent definition of breakfast is used, access to the School Breakfast Program does reduce the risk of skipping breakfast among low-income children, but not among higher income children (Devaney and Stuart 1998). On the other hand, Bhattacharya, Currie and Haider (2004) controlled for endogeneity by using a difference-in-differences approach based on changes in breakfast patterns during the school year and the summer, and found no evidence that children with access to the School Breakfast Program have a lower risk of skipping breakfast. Their approach, however, is potentially biased due to failure to account for the availability of summer food programs.

More recently, Waehrer (2007) used time use diary data from the Child Development Supplement of the Panel Study of Income Dynamics to estimate the impact of school breakfast participation on breakfast consumption, with the counter-intuitive finding that participation, as reported by parents, is linked to lower likelihood of children's breakfast consumption. However, results hinge on the assumption that breakfast consumption at schools is as accurately reported in time use diaries as is breakfast consumption at home—a problematic assumption given that fewer than 20 percent of the sample reported any meal consumption during the whole school day.

In short, existing research is inconclusive about whether access to the School Breakfast Program affects the likelihood that children eat breakfast, and if so, which children are most affected. The best evidence of a beneficial impact is from Devaney and Stuart (1998) and relies on data from 1992; the program has evolved considerably in size and form since that time. In this chapter, we examine the relationship between availability of the School Breakfast Program and the likelihood of skipping breakfast, using recent data collected from parents of elementary school children in Wisconsin. Our primary approach is to compare breakfast skipping among children with and without access to the program, controlling for other observable characteristics; we also consider instrumental variable models to control for unmeasured factors that may be correlated with program availability and breakfast skipping.

DATA

We use two primary sources of data in this chapter—the Early Childhood Longitudinal Survey—Kindergarten cohort (ECLS-K), and the Wisconsin Schools Food Security Survey. The former is used to examine School Breakfast Program participation patterns, as well as impacts on food insecurity; the latter is used to examine impacts on skipping breakfast, as the ECLS-K does not support that analysis.[1]

Early Childhood Longitudinal Survey-Kindergarten Cohort

Data are from the ECLS-K, wave 5 (third grade), restricted file. The ECLS-K is a nationally representative longitudinal survey providing information about children who entered kindergarten in the fall of 1998. A multistage probability sample design was employed to select the ECLS-K sample. Data were collected in the fall and the spring of kindergarten (1998-

99), the fall and spring of 1st grade (1999-2000), the spring of 3rd grade (2002), 5th grade (2004), and 8th grade (2007). A wide variety of information was collected from children, caregivers, and schools. Of particular relevance to this study, data collected from school administrators indicates whether the School Breakfast Program is offered, as well as key attributes of the program including where and at what time breakfast is served, as well as information on the share of children in the school eligible for free or reduced price meals. Relevant data collected from parents indicate, among other things, whether children usually eat school breakfast and/or school lunch, as well as the household's food security status using the standard 18-item food security scale. We use the restricted access data, which includes geographical identifiers; selected contextual data at the county level have been appended to the data. The sample for these analyses is limited to public school students for whom parents and school administrators provided survey responses during wave 5. Because of regulations related to the use of the restricted access data, all sample sizes reported, including subsamples, are rounded to the nearest ten.

Wisconsin Schools Food Security Survey

The Wisconsin Schools Food Security Survey is a self-administered survey sent home with students to parents of elementary school children in Wisconsin. It is used in this chapter to explore the relationship between school breakfast availability and children's breakfast patterns.

The survey includes a range questions about sources of food, participation in nutrition assistance programs, details about breakfast behavior including frequency of participating in school breakfast and skipping breakfast, reasons for not participating in school breakfast, food security based on the standard six-item scale, and demographic information. A variety of contextual data at the school, zipcode, and county levels have been appended to the data, including information on School Breakfast Program availability obtained from state records. Data were collected between fall of 2003 and fall of 2005.

Surveys were administered through a collaborative effort with University of Wisconsin – Extension. County Extension educators contacted local elementary schools regarding participation, worked with participating schools to ensure that surveys were disseminated using standard protocols, and coordinated local logistics. A total of 66 schools serving children in 26 counties participated during the primary survey period. For this chapter, we exclude 6 schools with ambiguous information about breakfast availability at school.[2] The sample size for this chapter consists of 7528 students. Note that the sample selection strategy was not designed to yield a fully representative sample of schools statewide, but rather, a sample of schools sufficiently diverse in terms of community attributes to allow identification of linkages between local attributes and outcomes of interest. Thus, overall prevalence rates of school meal participation should not be construed as representative of the state as a whole.

The mean response rate across schools was 69 percent, a high response rate for a self-administered survey. To assess the representativeness of the sample, we compared the share of surveys indicating that the child had received free or reduced price school meals in the past year with the official free and reduced price certification rate for the school, as provided by the Department of Public Instruction (DPI).[3] The average difference between the share reporting free or reduced-price meals and the official certification rate is minus two percentage points, and three-quarters of schools have reported rates within five percentage points of official rates, with official rates ranging from 9 percent to 80 percent of students.

DETERMINANTS OF PARTICIPATION IN THE SCHOOL BREAKFAST PROGRAM

In this section, we focus on participation in the School Breakfast Program, using the ECLS-K data. We introduce our analytic strategy, and present both descriptive and multivariate results.

Methods

Data are from the ECLS-K, as described above. For this analysis, the sample is limited to the subset of students who attend a school that participates in the School Breakfast Program, as our focus is on participation among students with access to the program. Information about whether the school participates in the program is available both from school administrators' and from parents' reports. Because there are some inconsistencies, we rely on administrators' reports, under the assumption that their information is most accurate, and that parents whose children do not participate may not, necessarily, know that the program is available. We exclude children for whom data from school administrators are not available.

It is possible that some of the schools in the sample offer universal free breakfast, whereby all children in the school are offered school breakfast at no cost regardless of income. We do not have an explicit indicator of this in the data; however, we identify 140 students who attend schools in which the free and reduced price eligibility rate for breakfast, as reported by school administrators, is 100 percent, and assume that this could be an indication of universal free breakfast, although we cannot be certain. Because availability of universal free breakfast would be expected to increase breakfast participation, and could potentially be correlated with other school-level variables of interest, we exclude these cases from the analysis, which does not significantly nor substantively affect the results.

We estimate probit models, where the dependent variable indicates whether the child usually eats a school breakfast, based on the parent's report.[4] This is coded as 1 if the parent responds in the affirmative to the question, "Does {Child} usually eat a breakfast provided by the school?". The conceptual model underlying this analysis reflects the expectation that participation in the School Breakfast Program is influenced by household characteristics that affect the perceived value of participating; programmatic and logistical factors that affect the ease of participating; and local norms regarding appropriate government roles and participation in assistance programs. As such, independent variables include household characteristics, programmatic characteristics, and contextual characteristics.

One set of independent variables includes household characteristics expected to reflect differences in need and/or preferences for participating. We include variables denoting household income, parental education, home ownership status, and number of children, as indicators of economic need; household structure cross-classified with employment, to capture the time constraints that may be present when parents work outside the home; estimated eligibility for free or reduced price meals, as participation may be more attractive when costs are lower; race and ethnicity, as participation in food assistance programs often varies across racial and ethnic groups; and gender, as some past work has found gender differences in school breakfast participation patterns.

A second set of independent variables includes programmatic and logistical factors that affect the ease of participation. We include an indicator for having breakfast served in the classroom, as compared to the cafeteria or other central location, as this may facilitate participation; the duration of the breakfast period, as longer periods may make the program more convenient; and the length of time between arrival at school and the start of classes, interacted with a dummy variable denoting children who take the school bus to school. For students who ride the bus, and for whom arrival time is thus exogenous to desired breakfast participation, arriving with more time before class is expected to make participation more feasible.

A third set of indicators is intended to proxy for local norms regarding appropriate government roles and participation in assistance programs. We include two measures—one intended to proxy for school norms regarding breakfast participation, and one intended to capture general liberal versus conservative tendencies in the community, which may be correlated with attitudes towards participating in government-sponsored food programs. For the former, we include the share of students in the school who are officially certified for free or reduced price meals. Higher certification rates denote a higher prevalence of low-income families, which may reduce any stigma associated with school breakfast participation—even for children who are not themselves low income. For the latter, we include the share of voters in the county who voted for the Democratic candidate in the 2004 presidential election, where local preference for Democrats versus Republicans serves as a proxy for a more positive attitude towards public assistance programs and is hypothesized to coincide with more openness to schools (as opposed to exclusively families) being involved in feeding schoolchildren. Because of the correlation between political preferences and economic conditions (as evidenced in these data), we also include a variable for median income based on the 2000 Census, as well as unemployment rate in the 12 months prior to the survey, both measured at the county level.

Finally, we include two sets of geographic indicators. We differentiate among regions, to identify areas where participation is more or less common than expected based on household characteristics. And, we include a series of variables describing the urban, surburban or rural character of the community. The ECLS-K provide an 8-part categorization including large cities, mid-size cities, large suburban areas, mid-size suburban areas, large towns, small towns, rural areas located within metropolitan statistical areas (MSAs), and rural areas outside of MSA's.

Results

How common is participation in the School Breakfast Program?

Participation in the School Breakfast Program is much less common than participation in the School Lunch Program. This reflects both differences in availability, as well as differences in participation when offered. In our broadest sample—third grade public school students with nonmissing survey data (regardless of breakfast availability)—35 percent of students usually eat school breakfast, as compared to 84 percent of students who usually eat school lunch (Table 1). Limiting the sample to children in schools where breakfast is offered—83 percent of the third graders for whom breakfast information is available from school administrators—42 percent usually eat school breakfast, compared to 82 percent who usually eat school lunch.[5] Looking more closely at participation in the two programs reveals that, unless students eat school lunch regularly, they are extremely unlikely to have any involvement with the breakfast program; but even among regular lunch participants, fewer than half participate in school breakfast.

Table 1. Participation in School Meal Programs, among Third Grade Public School Students

	N[1]	Percent Participating[2]	
		School Breakfast	School Lunch
All students[3]	10,350	35.3%	84.4%
Students in schools serving breakfast	6,680	41.8%	87.6%
Students who eat school lunch	5,610	43.0%	100%
Students who don't eat school lunch	890	6.8%	0%
Students who eat school breakfast	2,470	100%	97.6%
Students who don't eat school breakfast	4080	0%	79.5%

Note: Data are from the Early Childhood Longitudinal Survey—Kindergarten Cohort (ECLS-K), wave 5, restricted access file.

[1] Due to licensing requirements for ECLS-K restricted data, all sample sizes are rounded to the nearest 10.

[2] Percents are weighted.

[3] Full sample includes students with missing information on breakfast availability from school administrators.

Not only is school breakfast less widely utilized than school lunch, its use appears more skewed towards families at greatest risk of food-related hardships. As shown in Table 2, the prevalence of breakfast participation is closely related to income, declining steadily from almost three-quarters of students in the lowest income group to fewer than 10 percent in the highest-income group. In contrast, participation in school lunch decreases much less dramatically with income, from 97 percent to 72 percent. Consistent with this pattern, 80 percent of all children who eat school breakfast have meals that are either free or reduced price; among children who eat school lunch, far fewer—55 percent—eat meals that are free or reduced-price (not shown).

Table 2. Participation in School Meal Programs, by Household Characteristics

	N[1]	Percent Participating[2]	
		School Breakfast	School Lunch
Total (limited to children in schools serving school breakfast)	6,680	41.8%	87.6%
Income			
$15,000 or less	750	73.3%	96.8%
$15,001 to $20,000	430	64.2%	94.9%
$20,001 to $25,000	480	54.5%	94.9%
$25,001 to $30,000	550	52.9%	92.9%
$30,001 to $35,000	390	42.6%	92.0%
$35,001 to $40,000	510	40.2%	87.2%
$40,001 to $50,000	700	30.0%	83.6%
$50,001 to $75,000	1,090	19.5%	81.0%
$75,001 or more	1,050	9.3%	72.2%
Eligible for free or reduced price meals			
Eligible	2,800	59.8%	94.3%
Not eligible	3,160	20.7%	79.8%
Highest education in household			
Less than high school	770	70.0%	96.0%
High school	1,720	52.2%	93.1%
Some college	2,430	38.8%	86.7%
College degree	1,040	20.0%	81.6%
Graduate degree	710	14.5%	70.7%

Table 2. (Continued)

	N^1	Percent Participating[2]	
		School Breakfast	School Lunch
Number of children			
1	1,010	37.0%	88.0%
2	2,770	34.6%	84.4%
3	1,850	45.6%	89.5%
4 or more	1,060	58.4%	92.1%
Food security status			
Food secure	6,000	35.2%	85.4%
Food insecure	590	62.1%	95.7%
Region			
Northeast	980	30.5%	78.6%
Midwest	1,530	34.0%	89.6%
South	2,720	49.8%	89.4%
West	1,440	38.7%	87.6%
Urban vs. Rural Status			
Large city	1,030	43.2%	88.0%
Mid-size city	110	40.9%	87.3%
Large suburban area	1,400	3 5.3%	82.8%
Mid-size suburban area	440	35.0%	82.9%
Large town	250	46.6%	95.1%
Small town	530	45.1%	91.1%
Rural area in MSA	740	30.9%	84.0%
Rural area outside MSA	1,100	57.1%	94.7%

Note: Data are from the Early Childhood Longitudinal Survey—Kindergarten Cohort (ECLS-K), wave 5, restricted access file. Sample is limited to children in schools participating in School Breakfast Program.

[1] Due to licensing requirements for ECLS-K restricted data, all sample sizes are rounded to the nearest 10.

[2] Percents are weighted.

Examining other potential indicators of economic need, participation in school breakfast declines from 70 percent of students whose parents have less than a high school education to fewer than one-fifth of those with college-educated parents. And, participation increases sharply as the number of children in the household increases, from 37 percent of third graders in one-child households to 58 percent of those in households with four or more children. Focusing on food security, 62 percent of children who are food insecure eat school breakfast when it is available, as do only 35 percent of those who are food secure. (Of course, to the extent that school breakfast reduces the risk of food insecurity, the true underlying association between food insecurity and breakfast participation would be even stronger). School lunch participation, on the other hand, shows much more modest differences according to any of the various measures examined. Unlike the School Lunch Program, then, the School Breakfast Program appears to serve mostly, although not entirely, as a means of providing free or very low-cost meals to low income or at-risk children, as opposed to serving more broadly as a nutrition program for a cross- section of families.

School meal participation also differs across geographic areas, with sizable regional differences as well as differences among urban, suburban and rural areas. Participation is most common in the South, where just under half (49 percent) of children who have access to the School Breakfast Program participate, as compared to 39 percent in the west, 34 percent in the Midwest, and 31 percent in the northeast. In terms of urban-rural patterns, participation is most common in rural areas located out of metropolitan statistical areas (57 percent), lower in cities and towns (41-47 percent), still lower in the suburbs (35 percent), and lowest in rural areas that are part of MSAs (31 percent). In the case of school lunch, in contrast, there is substantially less geographic variation.

Multivariate Analysis of School Breakfast Program Participation

To assess factors predictive of participation in the School Breakfast Program, we estimate probit models with participation as the dependent variable, coded one to denote students who usually eat school breakfasts (based on parental report), and zero otherwise. Results are shown in Table 3.

The first panel focuses on household characteristics. Not surprisingly, participation declines as household income increases, and increases when there are more children in the household. There is no further impact of estimated eligibility for free or reduced price meals. In terms of household structure and employment, relative to two-parent households with one employed parent, participation is more likely among children with two employed parents in the household, perhaps reflecting the greater time constraints facing 2-parent households when both are employed. It also appears more likely among children with a single not-employed parent—a finding inconsistent with the time constraints hypothesis, and perhaps instead reflecting unmeasured hardship among the single unemployed households. Participation also becomes less common as parents' education level increases; education could proxy for earnings capacity and/or could be associated with different attitudes towards participation. And, participation is much more common among renters as compared to homeowners. There are large differences by race and ethnicity, with the probability of participation much higher among blacks, and to a lesser extent other racial and ethnic minorities, relative to whites. There are no significant differences in participation by gender.

The second panel focuses on geographic variables. Consistent with bivariate results, we find geographic differences—by region and by urban versus rural status—that persist even after controlling for differences in household characteristics. In particular, participation is more common in the Midwest and South relative to the Northeast, and is less common in cities and suburbs than in rural areas, net of other factors controlled for in the model.

Table 3. Probit Models of Participation in School Breakfast Program, Among Children Attending Schools that Offer Breakfast

	Model [1]		Model [2]	
	Coefficient	Standard Error	Coefficient	Standard Error
Intercept	0.164	0.237	0.056	0.240
Household Characteristics				
Income				
$15,000 or less	(omitted)		(omitted)	
$15,001 to $20,000	-0.170**	0.087	-0.169*	0.086
$20,001 to $25,000	-0.312***	0.085	-0.317***	0.085
$25,001 to $30,000	-0.320***	0.084	-0.333***	0.084
$30,001 to $35,000	-0.525***	0.094	-0.544***	0.094
$35,001 to $40,000	-0.388***	0.097	-0.409***	0.097
$40,001 to $50,000	-0.634***	0.104	-0.666***	0.104
$50,001 to $75,000	-0.716***	0.113	-0.731***	0.113
$75,001 or more	-0.957***	0.122	-0.961***	0.122
Eligible for free or reduced price meals				
Eligible	0.075	0.076	0.297***	0.103
Not eligible	(omitted)		(omitted)	
Number of children				
1	(omitted)		(omitted)	
2	0.032	0.057	0.037	0.057
3	0.192** *	0.061	0.201***	0.062
4 or more	0.417** *	0.071	0.423***	0.071
Household structure				
Single parent, not employed	0.198**	0.093	0.192**	0.093

Table 3. (Continued)

	Model [1]		Model [2]	
	Coefficient	Standard Error	Coefficient	Standard Error
Single parent, employed	0.062	0.063	0.05 8	0.063
2 parents, 1 employed	(omitted)		(omitted)	
2 parents, both employed	0.121**	0.048	0.123**	0.048
2 parents, neither employed	0.139	0.132	0.140	0.132
Other	0.252**	0.117	0.251**	0.118
Highest education in household				
Less than high school	(omitted)		(omitted)	
High school	-0.198***	0.066	-0.203***	0.066
Some college	-0.273***	0.066	-0.275***	0.066
College degree	-0.445***	0.082	-0.440***	0.082
Graduate degree	-0.639***	0.096	-0.629***	0.096
Housing arrangements				
Own home	(omitted)		(omitted)	
Rent home	0.214***	0.046	0.212***	0.046
Race				
White	(omitted)		(omitted)	
Black	0.639***	0.063	0.637***	0.063
Hispanic	0.350***	0.060	0.354***	0.060
Asian	0.192**	0.091	0.181*	0.092
Other	0.235** *	0.083	0.228***	0.083
Gender				
Male	(omitted)		(omitted)	
Female	-0.056	0.037	-0.056	0.037
Geographic Variables				
Region				
Northeast	(omitted)		(omitted)	
Midwest	0.280***	0.084	0.282***	0.085
South	0.284** *	0.081	0.284***	0.081
West	0.124	0.086	0.121	0.086
Urban vs. Rural Status				
Large city	-0.406***	0.080	-0.407***	0.079
Mid-size city	-0.318***	0.070	-0.308***	0.069
Large suburban area	-0.220***	0.070	-0.214***	0.069
Mid-size suburban area	-0.332***	0.089	-0.327***	0.089
Large town	-0.162	0.110	-0.159	0.108
Small town	-0.125	0.083	-0.134	0.082
Rural area in MSA	-0.271***	0.078	-0.282***	0.077
Rural area outside MSA	(omitted)		(omitted)	

Table 3. (Continued)

	Model [1]		Model [2]	
	Coefficient	Standard Error	Coefficient	Standard Error
Local Characteristics				
School free/reduced price meal certification rate	0.007***	0.001	0.010***	0.001
*School certification rate*child eligibility*			-0.005***	0.00 1
Percent of county voting democratic	-0.010***	0.002	-0.010***	0.002
Median income in county($100's)	-0.0012***	0.0003	-0.0012***	0.0003
Unemployment rate in county	0.006	0.0 14	0.005	0.0 14
Logistical & Programmatic Features				
Location of school breakfast served				
Cafeteria	(omitted)		(omitted)	
Classroom	0.504***	0.102	0.504***	0.102
Common areas	0.055	0.123	0.069	0.123
Other locations	-0.278	0.234	-0.268	0.234
Duration of school breakfast period(minutes)	0.004**	0.002	0.004**	0.002
Time between school arrival & start of class, for school bus riders				
Fewer than 10 minutes	(omitted)		(omitted)	
10 to 20 minutes	0.331***	0.072	0.325***	0.074
More than 20 minutes	0.938***	0.096	0.932***	0.096
Transportation to school				
School bus	(omitted)		(omitted)	
Parents drive	0.008	0.069	0.00 1	0.069
Carpool	0.051	0.149	0.044	0.149
Walk	0.138*	0.083	0.133	0.083
Someone else drives	-0.054	0.124	-0.060	0.124
Other	0.396**	0.190	0.400**	0.191
Log-likelihood	-3208.3 09		-3202.969	
N	6410		6410	

Notes: *=p<. 1, **=p<.05, ***=p<.01;

Data are from the Early Childhood Longitudinal Survey—Kindergarten Cohort (ECLS-K), wave 5, restricted access file.

Due to licensing requirements for ECLS-K restricted data, all sample sizes are rounded to the nearest 10. Dependent variable is school breakfast participation, coded 1 when the respondent indicates that the child usually eats a school breakfast.

Model also includes dummy variables denoting missing information on independent variables, wherever relevant, as well as variables for other housing arrangements.

The third panel focuses on local characteristics intended to reflect local norms. Even after controlling for household income and other characteristics, participation is significantly more common among children in schools with a larger share of low-income children (based on certification rates for free and reduced price meals). As noted, previous and current research find greater participation among lower-income households; we speculate that this translates into differing norms that influence participation rates, with greater participation in schools and communities in which it is more normative. Results are consistent with this pattern. We also examine differences according to local political preferences, expecting, as discussed previously, that participation would be more common in areas with democratic versus republican voting preferences; the former may have greater acceptance of the legitimacy of a public role in providing meals for children. Counter to our expectations, we found that participation actually decreases as democratic voting preferences increase, and this pattern is robust across a variety of model specifications. Because political preferences are highly correlated with economic attributes of communities, the model includes controls for median income and unemployment rate. We find no link between unemployment rate and breakfast participation, but a significant negative relationship between county median income and participation.

The fourth panel focuses on logistical and programmatic features that affect the convenience of participating in the School Breakfast Program. Results suggest that, indeed, such features are significantly linked to participation. First, the probability of participation increases dramatically when breakfast is served in the classroom rather than in the cafeteria. Second, the probability of participation increases with the duration of the breakfast period. Third, among the subset of students who take the bus to school, participation is more common as the time between arrival and the start of classes increases, that is, students are more likely to participate the more time they have available at school.

In Model 2, we also include an interaction between the school-level free and reduced- price certification rate and the child's free and reduced price eligibility status. The coefficient on child's eligibility status is now positive and significant, as is the certification rate, while the interaction is negative and significant. Thus, in schools with a small share of low-income children, a child's own eligibility status is a strong predictor of breakfast participation; in the context of a more sizable low-income student population, individual eligibility status becomes less important. To the extent that a higher certification rate proxies for reduced stigma, this suggests that, when participation is more normative due to a larger share of low-income children, children who themselves are not eligible for free or reduced price meals become increasingly likely to participate.

SCHOOL BREAKFAST PROGRAM AND FOOD INSECURITY

This section focuses on the relationship between the School Breakfast Program and food insecurity. As discussed earlier, the program could reduce food insecurity by providing children with a regular source of breakfast, in many cases free or at minimal cost, thereby both increasing the likelihood that children have food, and also freeing up family resources to feed others in the household.

Methods

We use the ECLS-K data, and limit the sample to low-income students, those below 185 percent of the poverty line. These are the students most at risk for food insecurity, and thus the group for which the program could potentially have a role in reducing food insecurity.

To estimate the impact of school breakfast on household food insecurity, we estimate a series of probit models with food insecurity as the dependent variable. We consider two measures of food insecurity: the official food security measure, based on an 18-item scale that classifies households as food secure or insecure based on the number of affirmative responses (with three or more affirmative responses required to be considered as food insecure); and a less restrictive measure, marginal food security, which we define as at least one affirmative response. This alternative measure has also been used in other research with the ECLS-K, and has been found to be a predictor of a variety of child outcomes (Jyoti, Frongillo, & Jones 2005; Winicki & Jemison 2003). We consider this less restrictive measure, in addition to the official measure, in part because of the unexpectedly low rate of food insecurity found in the ECLS-K sample relative to other national surveys (described below in our results). We also explored a measure of 'adult food insecurity'; results were quite similar to those for household food security and are not reported.

The key independent variable is the availability of the School Breakfast Program at the child's school. Other independent variables include a range of socioeconomic characteristics often predictive of food insecurity in past research, including income, parental education, race, household composition and employment, home ownership, and health status. We also include selected contextual characteristics including median rent (defined at the zipcode level), since higher housing costs have been linked to greater risk of food insecurity (Bartfeld and Dunifon 2006); as well as geographic region and indictors of urban, suburban, or rural character of the child's community, since past research reveals persistent geographic variation after controlling for household attributes. And, we control for the free and reduced price certification rate in the child's school, as the School Breakfast Program is more common in schools with larger share of low income children, although we do not anticipate that the certification rate would be predictive of food security outcomes after controlling for household income. The primary purpose of our model is to adequately control for differences between students with and without access to the program, so as to obtain an unbiased estimate of the impact of the School Breakfast Program.

By focusing on availability of school breakfast, rather than participation of a particular child, we address the policy question of whether making the program available—such that students may choose to participate based on their own needs and preferences—reduces the prevalence of food insecurity among students with access to the program. This avoids inherent selection problems stemming from the tendency of higher-need students to select into the program, a problem endemic to efforts to link voluntary participation in food assistance programs to measures of food-related hardship. The coefficient on breakfast availability indicates the average association between program availability and food insecurity, across all students with access to the program; to the extent that this association is causal, the impact of school breakfast on the subset of students who actually participate would, presumably, be greater.

Although focusing on availability rather than participation mitigates biases stemming from self-selection of students, there remain potential problems due to self-selection of schools into the program. While some states mandate participation for elementary schools, others only require participation when eligibility for free or reduced price meals (set at 185 percent of the poverty line) exceeds a given threshold, and still others leave the decision entirely up to schools or school districts. To the extent that schools with higher-risk students are more likely to offer breakfast, as suggested by the disproportionate availability of the program in schools with more low-income students, estimates of the impact of program availability on food security will be biased downward, unless underlying differences between students with and without access to the program are fully controlled for in the model.

To address this, we consider an instrumental variable approach. We use state-level mandates regarding the School Breakfast Program as instruments, and construct a dummy variable denoting whether each child's school is covered by a state mandate requiring that the program be offered. Seven states required that all public elementary schools offer breakfast during 2001; 16 states required that breakfast be offered when the free and reduced price certification rate exceeded a threshold that varied from 15 percent to 80 percent; and the remaining states had no requirement (FRAC 2003). We compared the school-reported certification rate to the relevant state policy to determine whether each child attended a school mandated to offer breakfast. We use the 'mandate' variable as an identifying variable in a probit model to predict breakfast availability, and use the predicted availability in our food security model. Implicit in this identification strategy is the assumption that the 'mandate' variable is uncorrelated with the error in the food security equation, that is, that the mandate variable is not associated with food security other than through its association with breakfast availability.

Although our main interest is in the impact of program availability on food insecurity, we also consider an alternative model that focuses on participation in the School Breakfast Program, as distinct from the availability of the program. For this analysis, we limit our sample to students in schools in which breakfast is offered (N=2620). Unfortunately, we do not have credible instruments for program participation that would allow us to control for unmeasured factors that may influence the participation decision.

Results

Descriptive results

Overall, 8.8 percent of children in our ECLS-K sample of third-graders who attend public schools live in households classified as food insecure, and 16.8 percent in households that are marginally food secure (Table 4). Note that the 'marginally food security' category also includes those classified as food insecure. The 8.8 percent food insecurity rate is considerably lower than expected, based on the official food security estimates generated by the Current Population Survey – Food Security Supplements. A Current Population Survey sample of children aged 7-9 during 2001-3, used as a comparison for the ECLS-K third grade sample used here, showed a household food insecurity rate of 19.3 percent--more than twice that in the ECLS-K sample.[6] The reason for this discrepancy is not apparent.

Food insecurity is strongly linked to income, in our sample and in other surveys. Here, we find that 16.6 percent of the low-income children (below 185 percent of the poverty line) in our sample are in households that are food insecure, as compared to 2.6 percent of higher income children. As a result, we limit our analysis to the low-income group; the extremely low rate of household food insecurity among higher income children makes it unlikely that the School Breakfast Program would have a meaningful or measurable impact. Note that a large majority of low-income children do have access to school breakfast; the relatively small number without access makes it more difficult to detect differences. Nonetheless, results show that the household food insecurity rate among low-income children with access to the School Breakfast Program is 16.1 percent, as compared to 24.5 percent among those without access; the analogous marginal food security rates are 29.2 percent and 42.2 percent.

Table 4. Household Food Insecurity among Third Grade Public School Students

	Total N[1]	Percent[2]	
		Standard Food Insecurity Measure	Marginal Food Security Measure
All students[3]	8,120	8.8%	16.8%
Below 185% poverty line	3,010	16.6%	30.1%
Above 185% poverty line	4,340	2.6%	6.1%
Limited to households below 185% of poverty line			
School offers breakfast	2,800	16.1%	29.2%
School doesn't offer breakfast	210	24.5%	42.2%

Notes: Data are from the Early Childhood Longitudinal Survey—Kindergarten Cohort (ECLS-K), wave 5, restricted access file.

Households are considered marginally food secure if the respondent answers at least one of the questions on the food security scale in the affirmative; the standard food security measure requires at least three affirmative responses to be considered food insecure.

[1] Due to licensing requirements for ECLS-K restricted data, all sample sizes are rounded to the nearest 10.

[2] Percents are weighted.

[3] Students with missing information on School Breakfast Program availability from school administrators are excluded.

Multivariate Analysis of School Breakfast Program and Food Insecurity

To assess the impact of school breakfast on household food insecurity, we estimate a probit model with food insecurity as the dependent variable (Table 5). We estimate an equivalent model for marginal food security, which uses a lower threshold to define food-related hardships. The key independent variable is a dummy variable denoting that the School Breakfast Program is available at the child's school. In the food insecurity model, the school breakfast coefficient is negative but not significant; in the marginal food security model, on the other hand, the coefficient is still negative, but larger in magnitude and highly significant (p<.01), suggesting reduced risk of marginal food security when the breakfast program is offered. Other variables in the model have coefficients largely in keeping with existing research on food security, with minor differences between the two models. The probability of household food insecurity declines as household income and education increase; is greater for renters as compared to homeowners; and increases with poorer health status and more children. In the standard food insecurity model we find no differences by race or ethnicity, net of other factors, other than a higher rate in the 'other race' category; however, blacks have significantly greater risk of marginal food security than do whites. We do not find significant differences according to household composition or employment status, with the exception of higher probability of marginal food security among children of single not-employed parents. Higher median rent is strongly associated with a heightened risk of food insecurity, though only weakly significant in the marginal food security model. Net of other factors we find little evidence of remaining regional differences in food insecurity, with the exception of a marginally significant higher probability of food insecurity in the West. Compared to rural areas, the risk of food insecurity is greater in small towns, mid-sized suburbs, and mid-sized cities, with only weak significance on any of these variables in the marginal food security model.

We use the coefficients from the marginal food security model to estimate the predicted probability of marginal household food security for a prototypical student, with and without access to the School Breakfast Program (Figure 1). Specifically, we consider a white student in the rural Midwest in a county with median rent of $600 per month, at a school with a 25 percent certification rate for free and reduced price meals; we assume the student is living with a single employed mother who is in good health, has a high school education, rents her home, has 2 children, and annual income of $15,001 - $20,000. In this case, the predicted probability of marginal food security is 47 percent if the school does not off breakfast, decreasing to 33 percent if breakfast is offered.

Table 5. Probit Models of Household Food Insecurity, among Low Income Third Grade Public School Students

	Standard Food Insecurity		Marginal Food Security	
	Coeff.	SE	Coeff.	SE
Intercept	-1.199***	0.257	-0.394*	0.223
School breakfast available	-0.113	0.123	-0.369***	0.107
Income				
$15,000 or less	(omitted)		(omitted)	
$15,001 to $20,000	-0.037	0.090	0.039	0.081
$20,001 to $25,000	-0.117	0.093	-0.164**	0.084
$25,001 to $30,000	-0.467***	0.107	-0.437***	0.091
$30,001 to $35,000	-0.358***	0.121	-0.411***	0.103
$35,001 to $40,000	-0.436***	0.139	-0.377***	0.115
$40,001 to $50,000	-0.526***	0.171	-0.531***	0.142
$50,001 to $75,000	-0.713	0.596	-0.697	0.465
	0	0	0	0
Highest education in household				
Less than high school	(omitted)		(omitted)	
High school	-0.156*	0.083	-0.127*	0.075
Some college	-0.187**	0.086	-0.123	0.076
College degree	-0.400***	0.145	-0.192*	0.118
Graduate degree	-0.675***	0.244	-0.452***	0.181
Housing arrangements				
Own	(omitted)		(omitted)	
Rent	0.169***	0.067	0.183***	0.059
Temporary	0.859**	0.414	0.342	0.409
Parent's health status				
Excellent	-0.186***	0.070	-0.153***	0.060
Good	(omitted)		(omitted)	
Poor	0.505***	0.077	0.401***	0.071
Number of children				
1	(omitted)		(omitted)	
2	0.045	0.112	0.064	0.098
3	0.155	0.112	0.164*	0.098
4 or more	0.247**	0.116	0.301***	0.102
Race of children				
White	(omitted)		(omitted)	
Black	0.073	0.094	0.234***	0.082

Table 4. (Continued)

	Standard Food Insecurity		Marginal Food Security	
	Coeff.	SE	Coeff.	SE
Hispanic	-0.076	0.091	0.024	0.080
Asian	0.015	0.139	0.021	0.122
Other	0.211*	0.120	0.234**	0.105
Household structure & employment				
Single parent, not employed	0.089	0.114	0.200**	0.103
Single parent, employed	-0.001	0.088	-0.076	0.078
2 parents, 1 employed	(omitted)		(omitted)	
2 parents, both employed	-0.113	0.08 1	-0.061	0.070
2 parents, neither employed	0.124	0.156	0.110	0.142
Other	-0.291	0.183	-0.225	0.158
Median rent	0.001**	0.0002	0.0003*	0.0002
Region				
Northeast	(omitted)		(omitted)	
Midwest	0.167	0.113	0.102	0.096
South	0.062	0.106	0.022	0.090
West	0.196*	0.108	0.139	0.094
Urban vs. Rural Status				
Large city	0.043	0.121	-0.103	0.102
Mid-size city	0.245**	0.113	0.164*	0.095
Large suburban	0.102	0.115	-0.029	0.097
Mid-size suburban	0.399***	0.137	0.184	0.121
Large town	0.238	0.175	-0.019	0.155
Small town	0.433***	0.126	0.183*	0.111
Rural area in MSA	0.159	0.137	0.086	0.115
Rural area outside MSA	(omitted)		(omitted)	
School free/reduced price meal certification rate	-0.001	0.001	-0.002	0.001
Log-likelihood	-1179.211		-1628.923	
N	2,960		2,960	

Notes: *=p<.1, **=p<.05, ***=p<.01

Data are from the Early Childhood Longitudinal Survey—Kindergarten Cohort (ECLS-K), wave 5, restricted access file.

Due to licensing requirements for ECLS-K restricted data, all sample sizes are rounded to the nearest 10. Households are considered marginally food secure if the respondent answers at least one of the questions on the food security scale in the affirmative; the standard food security measure requires at least three affirmative responses to be considered food insecure.

Model also includes dummy variables denoting missing information on independent variables, wherever relevant, as well as variables for other housing arrangements.

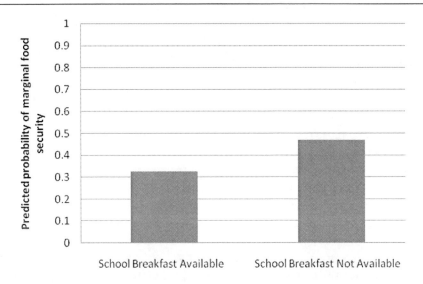

Figure 1. Predicted Probability of Marginal Household Food Security Among Low
Income Third Grade Public School Students, Based on Probit Model

To the extent that there are underlying differences between students with
and without access to school breakfast, beyond those controlled for in our
model, our estimates of program impact would be biased. To address this, we
use an instrumental variable approach to estimate the impact of School
Breakfast Program availability on food insecurity. As discussed earlier, we use
state-level mandates regarding the program as instruments. Table 6 shows our
first-stage model as well as the food insecurity models for both food security
measures, including predicted probability of breakfast availability as the key
independent variable.

Our first-stage model confirms that state policy mandates are indeed
strong and significant predictors of School Breakfast Program availability. Not
surprisingly, students whose school is covered by a state mandate to offer the
program are significantly more likely to have the program available at school
than are other students. Other predictors of breakfast availability include
region (most common in the south, and least common in the Midwest);
location (least common in surburban areas and large towns, and most common
in rural areas that are located within metropolitan areas); share of low-income
students in the school (with greater availability as share of low-income
students increases, though at a decreasing rate); and median housing costs (less
common in higher-rent areas). In the second-stage models, whether using the
standard or marginal food security measures, the coefficients on predicted

availability of the School Breakfast Program do not approach significance. We also considered an alternative operationalization of state mandates, by controlling for the level of the mandate rather than the applicability of the mandate to the particular child (that is, including separate variables to denote covering all elementary schools, elementary schools with at least a 75 percent free and reduced price meal certification rate, etc.). Results, not shown, are comparable to those reported.

Finally, we consider an alternative model in which student participation in the School Breakfast Program—as distinct from availability of the program at the school—is the key independent variable. As previously noted, our sample for this analysis is limited to the subset of students attending schools that offer breakfast. Results indicate that participation is associated with a significantly higher risk of food insecurity and marginal food security (Table 7), which we attribute to self-selection of higher risk children into the program. Unfortunately we do not have credible instruments that would allow us to control for unmeasured differences between participants and nonparticipants. The remaining variables in the model have similar associations with food insecurity and marginal security as found in our previous models.

SCHOOL BREAKFAST PROGRAM AND BREAKFAST SKIPPING: EVIDENCE FROM WISCONSIN

Methods

Our analysis relies on the Wisconsin Schools Food Security Survey, which asks parents, among other things, how many times their elementary school child skips breakfast in a typical school week. As with the food security analysis, we focus on availability of the School Breakfast Program, rather than on participation, thus examining how access to the program is linked to breakfast-skipping. We estimate a probit model with breakfast-skipping as the dependent variable, coded 1 if parents report that the child skips breakfast at least once in a typical week, otherwise coded 0. The key independent variable is the availability of the School Breakfast Program at the child's school, as reported by the Wisconsin Department of Public Instruction. Other independent variables include income, parental education, household composition and employment, home ownership, number of children, and degree of urbanicity (based on census data for the child's zipcode).

Table 6. Instrumental Variable Models of Household Food Insecurity, among Low Income Third Grade Public School Students

| | 1st Stage | | 2nd Stage | | | |
| | Prediction Model | | Standard Food Insecurity | | Marginal Food Security | |
	Coeff.	SE	Coeff.	SE	Coeff.	SE
Intercept	1.730 ***	0.310	-1.370***	0.348	-0.669**	0.300
Predicted probability of school breakfast availability			0.085	0.296	-0.133	0.254
Covered by State Policy Mandate	1.149***	0.159				
Region						
Northeast	(omitted)		(omitted)		(omitted)	
Midwest	-0.665***	0.140	0.185 (p=0.109)	0.115	0.121	0.098
South	1.108***	0.221	0.055	0.106	0.002	0.090
West	0.594***	0.159	0.193*	0.108	0.124	0.094
Urban vs. Rural Status						
Large city	0.135	0.217	0.043	0.121	-0.101	0.102
Mid-size city	0.088	0.206	0.244**	0.113	0.158*	0.095
Large suburban	-0.346**	0.171	0.118	0.116	-0.003	0.098
Mid-size suburban	-0.453**	0.203	0.406***	0.137	0.193 (p=0.109)	0.121
Large town	-0.833***	0.266	0.249	0.175	-0.006	0.154
Small town	0.101	0.223	0.433***	0.126	0.180 (p=0.106)	0.111
Rural area in MSA	0.396*	0.233	0.151	0.137	0.082	0.116

Table 6. (Continued)

| | 1st Stage | | 2nd Stage | | | |
| | Prediction Model | | Standard Food Insecurity | | Marginal Food Security | |
	Coeff.	SE	Coeff.	SE	Coeff.	SE
Rural area outside MSA	(omitted)		(omitted)		(omitted)	
School free/reduced price meal certification rate	0.038***	0.004	-0.003	0.003	-0.0002	0.003
Certification rate squared	-0.0002***	0.000	0.0000	0.0000	-0.0000	0.0000
Median rent in county	-0.003***	0.0004	0.001**	0.0003	0.0004**	0.0002
Highest education in household						
Less than high school	(omitted)		(omitted)		(omitted)	
High school	-0.193	0.182	-0.156*	0.083	-0.125*	0.075
Some college	-0.438***	0.174	-0.181**	0.086	-0.117	0.077
College degree	-0.396*	0.211	-0.391***	0.145	-0.182	0.118
Graduate degree	-0.267	0.281	-0.673***	0.244	-0.442***	0.180
Income						
$15,000 or less			(omitted)		(omitted)	
$15,001 to $20,000			-0.038	0.090	0.036	0.081
$20,001 to $25,000			-0.117	0.093	-0.163**	0.084
$25,001 to $30,000			-0.471***	0.107	-0.443***	0.091
$30,001 to $35,000			-0.363***	0.121	-0.419***	0.103
$35,001 to $40,000			-0.435***	0.139	-0.370***	0.115
$40,001 to $50,000			-0.525***	0.171	-0.529***	0.142
$50,001 to $75,000			-0.723	0.598	-0.735	0.465
$75,001 or more			0	0	0	0

Table 6. (Continued)

| | 1st Stage | | 2nd Stage | | | |
| | Prediction Model | | Standard Food Insecurity | | Marginal Food Security | |
	Coeff.	SE	Coeff.	SE	Coeff.	SE
Housing ownership						
Own			(omitted)		(omitted)	
Rent			0.167***	0.067	0.174***	0.058
Temporary			0.870**	0.415	0.374	0.412
Parent's health status						
Excellent			-0.187***	0.070	-0.154***	0.060
Good			(omitted)		(omitted)	
Poor			0.506***	0.077	0.403***	0.071
Number of children						
1			(omitted)		(omitted)	
2		0.047	0.112	0.068	0.097	0.097
3		0.157	0.112	0.167*	0.098	0.098
4 or more		0.247**	0.116	0.303***	0.102	
Race of children						
White			(omitted)		(omitted)	
Black		0.073	0.094	0.232***	0.082	
Hispanic		-0.079	0.091	0.021	0.080	
Asian		0.014	0.139	0.015	0.122	
Other		0.212*	0.120	0.227***	0.105	
Household structure & employment						
Single parent, not employed		0.090	0.114	0.204**	0.103	

Table 6. (Continued)

	1st Stage		2nd Stage			
	Prediction Model		Standard Food Insecurity		Marginal Food Security	
	Coeff.	SE	Coeff.	SE	Coeff.	SE
Single parent, employed		0.002	0.088	-0.064	0.078	
2 parents, 1 employed	(omitted)		(omitted)			
2 parents, both employed		-0.110	0.081	-0.050	0.069	
2 parents, neither employed		0.128	0.156	0.117	0.142	
Other		-0.290	0.184	-0.211	0.158	
Log-likelihood	-408.939	-1179.572		-1634.612		
N	2,960	2,960		2,960		

Notes: $*=p<.1$, $**=p<.05$, $***=p<.01$

Data are from the Early Childhood Longitudinal Survey—Kindergarten Cohort (ECLS-K), wave 5, restricted access file.

Due to licensing requirements for ECLS-K restricted data, all sample sizes are rounded to the nearest 10. Households are considered marginally food secure if the respondent answers at least one of the questions on the food security scale in the affirmative; the standard food security measure requires at least three affirmative responses to be considered food insecure.

Model also includes dummy variables denoting missing information on independent variables, wherever relevant, as well as variables for other housing arrangements.

Table 7. Probit Models of Household Food Insecurity, among Low Income Third Grade Public School Students with Access to School Breakfast Program

	Standard Food Insecurity		Marginal Food Security	
	Coeff.	SE	Coeff.	SE
Intercept	-1.438***	0.249	-0.935***	0.215
Participates in School Breakfast	0.144**	0.070	0.197***	0.061
Income				
$15,000 or less	(omitted)		(omitted)	
$15,001 to $20,000	-0.019	0.095	0.081	0.085
$20,001 to $25,000	-0.084	0.100	-0.099	0.089
$25,001 to $30,000	-0.484***	0.116	-0.479***	0.099
$30,001 to $35,000	-0.331***	0.132	-0.406***	0.114
$35,001 to $40,000	-0.461***	0.155	-0.444***	0.128
$40,001 to $50,000	-0.448**	0.200	-0.699***	0.175
$50,001 to $75,000	-5.412	4830.308	-0.694	0.557
$75,001 or more	0	0	0	0
Highest education in household				
Less than high school	(omitted)		(omitted)	
High school	-0.156*	0.087	-0.110	0.078
Some college	-0.189**	0.091	-0.116	0.081
College degree	-0.477***	0.169	-0.227*	0.135
Graduate	-0.621 **	0.273	-0.402**	0.207
Housing ownership				
Own	(omitted)		(omitted)	
Rent	0.145**	0.072	0.120*	0.063
Temporary	1.035**	0.443	0.460	0.437
Parent's health status				
Excellent	-0.155**	0.076	-0.130**	0.065
Good	(omitted)		(omitted)	
Poor	0.498***	0.082	0.386***	0.075
Number of children				
1	(omitted)		(omitted)	
2	-0.009	0.119	0.043	0.104
3	0.125	0.118	0.186*	0.104
4 or more	0.245**	0.124	0.330***	0.109
Race of children				
White	(omitted)		(omitted)	
Black	0.035	0.100	0.196**	0.087
Hispanic	-0.059	0.098	0.047	0.086

Table 7. (Continued)

	Standard Food Insecurity		Marginal Food Security	
	Coeff.	SE	Coeff.	SE
Asian	-0.119	0.169	-0.004	0.144
Other	0.025*	0.140	0.045	0.120
Household structure & employment				
Single parent, not employed	0.077	0.119	0.176*	0.108
Single parent, employed	-0.006	0.095	-0.08 8	0.084
2 parents, 1 employed	(omitted)		(omitted)	
2 parents, both employed	-0.101	0.088	-0.092	0.075
2 parents, neither employed	0.175	0.165	0.099	0.152
Other	-0.295	0.192	-0.194	0.165
Median rent	0.001*	0.0003	0.0004	0.0002
Region				
Northeast	(omitted)		(omitted)	
Midwest	0.201 (p=108)	0.125	0.131	0.107
South	0.072	0.114	-0.003	0.098
West	0.142	0.119	0.027	0.104
Urban vs. Rural Status				
Large city	0.158	0.132	-0.065	0.112
Mid-size city	0.319***	0.123	0.207**	0.103
Large suburban	0.161	0.128	0.012	0.107
Mid-size suburban	0.485***	0.151	0.269**	0.133
Large town	0.271	0.187	-0.048	0.166
Small town	0.530***	0.136	0.259**	0.119
Rural area in MSA	0.211	0.147	0.128	0.124
Rural area outside MSA	(omitted)		(omitted)	
School free/reduced price meal certification rate	-0.001	0.001	-0.001	0.001
Log-likelihood	-1016.068		-1392.186	
N	2,620		2,620	

Notes: *=p<.1, **=p<.05, ***=p<.01

Data are from the Early Childhood Longitudinal Survey—Kindergarten Cohort (ECLS-K), wave 5, restricted access file.

Due to licensing requirements for ECLS-K restricted data, all sample sizes are rounded to the nearest 10. Households are considered marginally food secure if the respondent answers at least one of the questions on the food security scale in the affirmative; the standard food security measure requires at least three affirmative responses to be considered food insecure.

Model also includes dummy variables denoting missing information on independent variables, wherever relevant, as well as variables for other housing arrangements.

Breakfast-skipping differs from food insecurity in that it occurs at nontrivial levels in all income groups. As such, we do not limit our analysis to a low-income sample. We hypothesize that school breakfast may moderate the relationship between income and breakfast-skipping, however, and explore this by estimating a model with interactions between income and breakfast availability.

Finally, we consider an instrumental variable model. Unlike in our analysis of breakfast availability and food insecurity, we cannot rely on state policy variables as instruments, as our sample is limited to Wisconsin. Instead we use the free and reduced price meal certification rate (and rate squared), in the school, as well as median rent (from the 2000 Census, defined at the zipcode level), as identifying variables in a probit model of breakfast availability. Consistent with the ECLS-K analysis, we expect the availability of school breakfast to differ between low- income and higher-income schools, and between wealthier and less wealthy communities (as captured by differences in housing costs), yet we do not expect these school and community indicators to directly impact breakfast-skipping patterns after controlling for household characteristics.

Results

Breakfast-skipping among children with and without access to the School Breakfast Program

Overall, 24 percent of parents report that their child skips breakfast at least once in a typical school week, with 9 percent reporting 3 or more times. Breakfast skipping patterns are similar in schools with and without the School Breakfast Program—23.7 vs 24.8 percent (Table 7). Direct comparisons between breakfast patterns in schools with and without breakfast are complicated by substantial differences among the students in the two groups of schools. In the Wisconsin Schools sample used here, 44 of 59 schools offer breakfast. The School Breakfast Program schools serve, on average, a disproportionately low income population: the average free and reduced price meal eligibility rate among breakfast-providing schools in the sample is .47, as compared to .26 among the non-breakfast schools (not shown). As such, comparisons of meal patterns are more informative when they differentiate between meal-skipping among higher-risk versus lower-risk students.

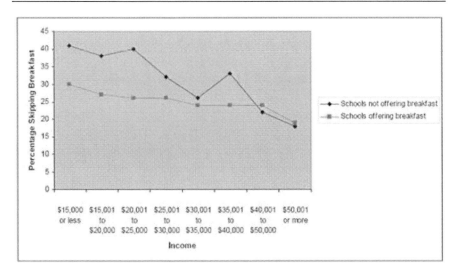

Figure 2. Breakfast-Skipping among Elementary School Children in Wisconsin, by
Income Level and School Breakfast Program Availability

Table 8. Breakfast-Skipping among Wisconsin Elementary School Students

	N	*Percent skipping breakfast*	
		Children with School Breakfast Available	Children without School Breakfast Available
Total	7,428	23.7%	24.8%
Food security status			
Food insecure	1,630	35.2%	46.1%
Food secure	5,898	20.3%	20.1%
Food pantry use			
Yes	905	30.2%	45.7%
No	6,524	22.6%	22.7%
Food stamp participation			
Yes	1,101	28.6%	37.2%
No	6,335	22.6%	23.4%

Note: Data are from the Wisconsin Schools Food Security Survey.
Students are considered to skip breakfast if the respondent indicates that the child skips
breakfast at least once in a typical week.

Figure 2 illustrates the prevalence of breakfast-skipping among various income groups, looking separately at students in schools that do and do not offer breakfast. The rate of skipping is much more strongly linked to income in the non-breakfast schools. In those schools, the prevalence of breakfast-skipping ranges from 38 to 41 percent in the three lowest income groups, from 26 to 33 percent in the three higher groups, and from 18 to 19 percent in the highest income groups. In the breakfast schools, on the other hand, breakfast skipping is much less variable across groups, and rates are sharply lower than in the non-breakfast schools at the lower income levels. Simple descriptive statistics, then, suggest that the availability of school breakfast may reduce the differential risk of skipping breakfast that is evident among lower income children.

Table 8 compares the prevalence of breakfast-skipping in breakfast and non-breakfast schools, according to a variety of other household attributes suggestive of economic need. Specifically, we look at breakfast-skipping in families classified as food insecure versus secure; who use food pantries versus who do not; and who receive food stamps versus not. When school breakfast isn't available, almost half of children in food insecure households skip breakfast at least once in a typical week (46.1 percent); this falls to 35.2 percent among children whose school participates in the program. Among children in food secure households, the rate of breakfast-skipping is approximately 20 percent regardless of school breakfast availability. A similar pattern holds when stratifying by use of food pantries: Among children without access to school breakfast, 45.7 percent of those who live in households that have received food from food pantries in the past year skip one or more breakfasts in a typical week, as compared to 30.2 percent of pantry users in schools that offer breakfast. Among children whose families have not used food pantries, the rate of breakfast skipping is approximately 23 percent regardless of breakfast availability. Stratifying by food stamp use also tells a similar story. In sum, the descriptive data provide preliminary evidence that availability of school breakfast is associated with lower likelihood of skipping breakfast among vulnerable subsets of elementary school students, and thus reduces the gap in breakfast-skipping between more vulnerable and less vulnerable children.

Multivariate Analysis of School Breakfast Program and Breakfast-Skipping

To more formally estimate the impact of the School Breakfast Program on the probability that a child skips breakfast, we turn to a multivariate approach, considering several different models. First, we estimate a probit model with a dichotomous measure of breakfast-skipping as the dependent variable, and the key independent variable an indicator of the availability of the breakfast program (Table 9). Other variables include a variety of household characteristics broadly reflective of economic wellbeing, which may also be linked to breakfast patterns.

Table 9. Probit Models of Breakfast-Skipping among Elementary School Children in Wisconsin

	Model 1		Model 2		Model 3	
	Coeff.	SE	Coeff.	SE	Coeff.	SE
Intercept	-0.367**	0.186	-0.444**	0.188	-0.301	0.190
School breakfast available	-0.105***	0.038	0.031	0.054		
Predicted probability of school breakfast availability[1]					-0.153***	0.057
Income						
$15,000 or less	0.242***	0.066	0.509***	0.119	0.249***	0.067
$15,001 to $20,000	0.183***	0.069	0.453***	0.123	0.191***	0.070
$20,001 to $25,000	0.190***	0.074	0.517***	0.142	0.182**	0.075
$25,001 to $30,000	0.164**	0.079	0.301*	0.167	0.195**	0.081
$30,001 to $35,000	0.103	0.065	0.167	0.114	0.101	0.066
$35,001 to $40,000	0.184***	0.062	0.385***	0.110	0.191***	0.063
$40,001 to $50,000	0.112*	0.067	0.091	0.124	0.121*	0.068
$50,001 or more	(omitted)		(omitted)		(omitted)	
*Breakfast availability*Income*						
Available*$15,000 or less			-0.349***	-0.349		
Available*$15,001 to $20,000			-0.374***	-0.374		
Available*$20,001 to $25,000			-0.443***	-0.443		
Available*$25,001 to $30,000			-0.197	-0.197		
Available*$30,001 to $35,000			-0.104	-0.104		
Available*$35,001 to $40,000			-0.297**	-0.297		
Available*$40,001 to $50,000			0.015	0.015		
Available*$50,001 or more			(omitted)			
Housing arrangements						
Own	(omitted)		(omitted)		(omitted)	
Rent	0.083*	0.043	0.083*	0.043	0.076*	0.044

Table 9. (Continued)

	Model 1		Model 2		Model 3	
	Coeff.	SE	Coeff.	SE	Coeff.	SE
Homeless	-0.033	0.156	-0.023	0.156	-0.070	0.168
Highest education in household						
Less than high school	(omitted)		(omitted)		(omitted)	
High school	-0.054	0.082	-0.052	0.082	-0.053	0.084
Some college	-0.122	0.082	-0.119	0.082	-0.128	0.084
College degree	-0.312***	0.086	-0.312***	0.086	-0.322***	0.087
Household structure						
Single mother, not employed	-0.045	0.106	-0.05 1	0.107	-0.028	0.108
Single mother, employed	0.149**	0.060	0.142**	0.060	0.144**	0.061
Single father	0.013	0.103	0.011	0.103	0.014	0.104
2 parents, 1 employed	(omitted)		(omitted)		(omitted)	
2 parents, both employed	0.03 8	0.047	0.03 8	0.047	0.025	0.047
2 parents, neither employed	0.008	0.131	0.010	0.131	0.010	0.133
Grandparents	0.006	0.151	0.000	0.151	0.042	0.156
Other	0.138*	0.077	0.141*	0.077	0.108	0.078
Number of children						
1	(omitted)		(omitted)		(omitted)	
2	-0.032	0.045	-0.038	-0.038	-0.04	.045
3	-0.006	0.050	-0.005	-0.005	-0.011	.050
4 or more	0.034	0.061	0.031	0.031	0.027	.062
Urban vs. Rural Status of zipcode						
All urban	(omitted)		(omitted)		(omitted)	
Mostly urban	-0.326**	0.155	-0.330**	0.155	-0.339**	0.156
Mostly rural	-0.201	0.158	-0.208	0.158	-0.215	0.158
All rural	-0.251	0.155	-0.260*	0.155	-0.252	0.155
Log-likelihood	-4059.274		-4048.727		-3938.127	
N	7528		7528		7299	

Notes: *=p<.1, **=p<.05, ***=p<.01

Data are from the Wisconsin Schools Food Security Survey.

The dependent variable, breakfast-skipping, is coded as 1 if the respondent indicates that the child skips breakfast at least once in a typical week,Model also includes dummy variables denoting missing information on independent variables, wherever relevant.

[1] Predictions generated by probit model of School Breakfast Program availability; model shown in Table 10.

Results suggest that the availability of school breakfast significantly reduces the probability of breakfast-skipping (p<.01). Skipping breakfast is also more common among children from lower income households and those living in households that rent versus own their home, and less common among children with a college-educated parent. Education may proxy here for economic resources, or may be associated with greater awareness of the importance of breakfast for children. And, skipping breakfast is more common among children living with a single employed mother, relative to those living with both an employed and an at-home parent, perhaps reflecting time constraints that may make it more difficult for single employed parents to consistently feed children breakfast before school. There are no significant differences according to the number of children, and some evidence of less breakfast-skipping in mixed urban-rural communities (specifically, communities that are predominantly but not fully urban) as compared to fully urban communities.

In our next model, we look more closely at the role of the School Breakfast Program, allowing for different impacts among children at greater versus lesser risk. Specifically, we include, in addition to a breakfast program indicator, a series of interaction terms between breakfast program availability and income group. We expect that, rather than a constant impact, access to the School Breakfast Program may moderate the risk associated with low income. Results are consistent with this hypothesis. The income coefficients are highest for the lowest income group, and decline as income increases, indicating the relationship between income and breakfast-skipping in the absence of the program. The interaction terms on the several lowest income categories are negative and highly significant, suggesting that availability of school breakfast offsets the higher risk of breakfast-skipping found among the lower income groups. When breakfast is offered at school, then, income appears to be much less important an influence on breakfast consumption.

In our third and final model, we use an instrumental variable strategy to control for unmeasured differences between children with and without access to breakfast at school. As discussed earlier, the identifying variables are the share of children in the school who are certified for free or reduced price meals (and the rate squared), as well as the median rent. Schools with a larger share of low-income students are much more likely to offer school breakfast, while the share of low-income children is not expected to be linked to breakfast patterns at the individual level, net of household income and other characteristics. Likewise, we expect wealthier areas, proxied by higher housing costs, to be less likely to offer school breakfast, but we do not posit any direct link between housing costs and breakfast skipping. The first-stage model, shown in Table 10, confirms that the certification rate is indeed a strong predictor of breakfast availability (at a decreasing rate, as evidenced by the negative coefficient on the squared term). Other predictors of access to school breakfast include lower median rent in the area, and living in a more urban area. In the second-stage model, the predicted probability of breakfast availability is negatively and significantly linked to breakfast skipping. Results are consistent with our earlier model, which controls for actual rather than predicted availability. We also examined whether results were sensitive to our choice of identifying variables, by alternately including one or the other of the potential identifying variables in the breakfast skipping model as well as in the prediction model. While the impact is most precisely estimated when certification rate and median rent are both used to identify the model, as in the results shown, we find a significant impact of school breakfast with either one serving as an identifying restriction. In general, results of the instrumental variable model appear robust to a variety of specifications.

Table 10. Probit Model of School Breakfast Availability among Elementary School Children in Wisconsin[1]

	Coeff.	SE
Intercept	0.931***	0.062
School free/reduced price certification rate	3.101***	0.132
School certification rate squared	-1 .972***	0.154
Median rent($100's)	-0.179***	0.006
Urban vs. Rural Status		
All urban	(omitted)	
Mostly urban	-0.253***	0.03 8
Mostly rural	-0.260** *	0.039
All rural	-0.259***	0.039
Log-likelihood	-1992.428	
N	7553	

Notes: *=p<.1, **=p<.05, ***=p<.01

Data are from the Wisconsin Schools Food Security Survey.

Model also includes dummy variables denoting missing information on independent variables, wherever relevant.

[1] Model is used to estimate the predicted probability of school breakfast availability in Model 3, Table 9.

To illustrate the magnitude of the estimated impact of school breakfast, we use the coefficients from Model 2 in Table 9 to estimate the predicted probability of skipping breakfast for prototypical students at varying income levels, with and without access to the School Breakfast Program (Table 11). Specifically, we consider a student in a rural area, who is living with a two employed parents with a high school education, in a household with 2 children and a rented home, at each of eight different income levels. In the absence of the School Breakfast Program, the predicted probability of skipping breakfast at least once per week is strongly linked to income, declining from a high of .42 at the lowest income level to a low of .25 at the highest income level. In contrast, when the School Breakfast Program is available, the additional risk associated with low income declines dramatically, with the predicted probabilities ranging from a high of .30 at the lowest income to a low of .24 at the highest income. Consistent with the earlier descriptive results (Figure 2), predictions derived from the multivariate analysis indicate that access to the School Breakfast Program sharply reduces the negative relationship that otherwise exists between low income and breakfast-skipping.

**Table 11. Predicted Probability of Breakfast-Skipping among
Wisconsin Elementary School Students with and without
Access to School Breakfast Program**

	Predicted probability of skipping breakfast	
N	Children with School Breakfast Available	Children without School Breakfast Available
Income		
$15,000 or less	.30	.42
$15,001 to $20,000	.27	.40
$20,001 to $25,000	.27	.42
$25,001 to $30,000	.28	.34
$30,001 to $35,000	.27	.29
$35,001 to $40,000	.28	.37
$40,001 to $50,000	.28	.27
$50,000 or more	.25	.24

Note: Predicted probabilities are based on probit model of breakfast skipping, using data from the Wisconsin Schools Food Security Survey (see Table 9, Model 2). Predictions assume the student's household has 2 children and 2 employed parents, with high school education, rents their home, and lives in rural area in Wisconsin.

CONCLUSION

This chapter provides an updated look at patterns and determinants of School Breakfast Program participation, as well as impacts of the program on food insecurity and on breakfast skipping. Past research clearly shows that school breakfast is inconsistently available, and when available, inconsistently implemented, with widely ranging participation patterns. This matters more, to the extent that offering the program, and encouraging participation, is in fact beneficial to children. In this chapter, we confirm that participation is inconsistent, even among children who appear to have unmet food-related needs, and we identify a range of factors at the household and school levels that appear important in influencing the decision to participate. And, we provide evidence that access to the program is beneficial in at least two ways—enhancing food security and reducing the likelihood that children skip breakfast on school days, with more robust findings for the latter outcome. Many would consider these outcomes desirable in their own right; they are particularly important in light of growing evidence of their links to both cognitive and health-related outcomes including, for instance, academic performance and obesity (see, e.g., Joyoti, Frongillo, and Jones 2005; Haines et al 2007).

Our analysis confirms that school breakfast is much less widely used than school lunch, even among children with access to both programs. Furthermore, breakfast participation is almost entirely limited to a subset of the students who regularly eat school lunch. The program appears to serve as an expanded way of utilizing school meals for a subset of the students already predisposed to such meals; it receives only extremely limited use among other students. And, in contrast to school lunch, school breakfast appears to be used primarily by the subset of students who are most vulnerable. At the same time, there remains a substantial share of at-risk children who have access to the program yet do not participate—including 38 percent of those who are food insecure.

Multivariate analyses suggest that both economic vulnerability and time constraints are linked to participation, with low income and education, more children, and having two employed parents in the home emerging as significant predictors. We also find indirect evidence that local norms may be important in the participation decision, as evidenced by significantly higher participation in schools with a larger share of low-income students, as well as in neighborhoods with lower median incomes. Furthermore, it appears the normative nature of participation in low-income schools may have spillover effects on higher income children who might otherwise be less inclined to participate. Pronounced differences in participation according to race and ethnicity could also reflect differences in norms or preferences. On the other hand, and counter to our expectation, we found less likelihood of participation among children living in counties with more liberal political climates, suggesting that prevailing wisdom about political norms and attitudes towards public programs may not be reflected in school meal program decisions.

Of particular interest, we found that programmatic and logistical aspects of how breakfast is structured at the school are significantly linked to the likelihood of participation. Results strongly support the hypothesis that increasing the convenience of the School Breakfast Program leads to greater participation, with evidence of the importance of where breakfast is offered (classroom versus cafeteria), the duration of the breakfast period, and the arrival time of buses relative to the start of classes. While smaller-scale local studies have found evidence that features such as in-class breakfast increase participation (see, e.g., Lent and Emerson 2006; Wong and Emerson 2007), this is the first evidence, to our knowledge, of its impact on a national scale.

Understanding factors that facilitate or impede participation in the School Breakfast Program is particularly important to the extent that participation contributes to desirable outcomes for children. Our preferred analyses avoid an explicit focus on participation impacts, due to fairly intractable problems stemming from self-selection of more vulnerable children into the program, instead capitalizing on differences in program availability to assess program impacts.

Our findings suggest that school breakfast availability is linked to a lower probability of marginal household food security among low-income children, though not to food insecurity at the standard threshold. That is, the program appears beneficial in offsetting food-related concerns among at-risk families, though not necessarily in alleviating food insecurity once hardships have crossed the food insecurity threshold. The magnitude of the estimated impact is substantial, with availability of school breakfast reducing the predicted probability of marginal food security from 47 percent to 33 percent in the hypothetical case considered here. It is notable that food insecurity at this marginal threshold has also been linked to poor developmental trajectories for children (Jyoti, Frongillo, and Jones 2005). While it is possible that unmeasured differences between schools that do and do not offer the program could bias our results, we find it more plausible that any bias would result in underestimates, rather than overestimates, of the true impact, given that school breakfast is disproportionately offered in schools with higher-need populations, at least based on observable characteristics. On the other hand, we were unable to substantiate our findings with an instrumental variable model, despite the existence of a strong state policy instrument. We note the relatively small number of low-income students in our sample who do not have access to school breakfast, thus hampering our ability to obtain more precise estimates of program impact.

In contrast to a negative association between School Breakfast Program availability and marginal food security, we found a positive association between actual participation in the program and both of the food insecurity outcomes. We attribute this relationship to self- selection of higher risk children into the program; that is, we expect that children with more immediate food security concerns would be more likely to eat a school breakfast when available, making it difficult to obtain valid impact estimates. This problem is pervasive in the literature on food assistance program participation and food insecurity. Overall, we find the analyses that focus on availability of the program, rather than participation, to have both greater policy relevance and greater statistical merit.

Evidence that availability of the School Breakfast Program reduces the risk of breakfast- skipping is robust. Results, which are based on Wisconsin data, suggest that offering breakfast significantly reduces the probability of skipping at least one breakfast per week, and that offering breakfast at school serves to moderate the risk of breakfast-skipping associated with low income. A beneficial impact is also evident when we use an instrumental variable approach, further strengthening our confidence in the findings. Our results are broadly consistent with those of Devaney & Stuart (1998), though we use much more recent data, look more formally at how impacts change across income levels, and use an instrumental variable approach as a robustness check. Note that these results are based on data for only one state; it is possible that the impact of the program on breakfast-skipping might differ elsewhere, particularly if patterns of program uptake vary across locations.

Taken as a whole, our findings indicate that access to the School Breakfast Program yields significant benefits in terms of enhancing food security among families at the margin of food insecurity, and increasing the probability that children—particularly low-income children— eat breakfast in the morning. Currently, the share of schools that offer the program ranges dramatically across states, from a low of 51.5 percent of schools offering lunch in Connecticut, to availability in more than 95 percent of schools in 13 states (FRAC 2007). Our findings suggest that making school breakfast more broadly available would be beneficial in ensuring that more children start their school day with a meal, and that fewer families are confronted with uncertain access to sufficient food.

Furthermore, our findings on participation patterns suggest that these benefits could also be enhanced with greater participation among children who already have access to the program.

On the one hand, the most vulnerable children are already the most likely to participate, suggesting that the program is generally well targeted. At the same time, there appears to be substantial unmet need, as evidenced by nontrivial amounts of nonparticipation among children who are food insecure and/or who don't consistently eat breakfast. As such, it seems likely that strengthening participation could yield further benefits, though likely at decreasing rates. To the extent that stigma, negative impressions of school breakfast, or logistical barriers are dampening participation among children who would find it beneficial to participate, identifying and taking steps to counter such barriers seems warranted.

Our results point to potential strategies to enhance participation through program design as well as outreach efforts. In particular, the relationship between program attributes and participation patterns suggest that there are policy levers that can be used to enhance participation by removing logistical barriers. For instance, Kansas mandates that all school buses arrive at school with adequate time for children to eat breakfast (FRAC 2007); in Milwaukee, all schools that participate in a Universal Free Breakfast program are required to make breakfast available in the classroom.

In terms of program outreach, the concentration of participants among the subset of students who regularly eat lunch suggests that outreach efforts may be most effective if they market school breakfast as an expansion of the school lunch concept, building on students' connection with that program. In addition, participation patterns suggest that expanding school breakfast to additional schools may be most effective as a means to increase participation in schools that already have relatively high rates of lunch participation, as students in those schools are most likely to be receptive to the breakfast program. Efforts to expand the reach of school breakfast to a broader cross-section of students may benefit by outreach/marketing strategies that focus on convenience or other potential benefits, in addition to the economic benefits of participating, to help broaden the appeal beyond the current primarily low-income clientele. To the extent that stigma associated with the program may discourage participation, successfully targeting a broader cross-section may also help to counter existing stereotypes. Social marketing efforts to present the program as normative would likely be effective.

A variety of extensions to this work would be of value. First, it would be useful to examine how individual participation in the School Breakfast Program changes over time; the ECLS-K is well suited to this given the longitudinal structure of the data. Likewise, it could be beneficial to examine the relationship between the School Breakfast Program and food security in a longitudinal framework, although the relatively low rates of food insecurity in the ECLS-K could create some challenges for such an analysis. Although not directly related to the School

Breakfast Program, the unexpectedly low rate of food insecurity found in these data is also a topic that warrants further attention, particularly given the potential value of the data to explore the relationship between food insecurity and a variety of child outcomes. In terms of the relationship between the School Breakfast Program and breakfast skipping, it would be useful to attempt to replicate these findings with data from a national sample; unfortunately, the ECLS-K are not well suited to this as breakfast skipping cannot be accurately identified.

Finally, we note some inherent limitations in our data. With regard to school breakfast participation, we only have information on parents' report of whether a child 'usually eats a breakfast provided by the school'. We do not know anything about occasional (rather than usual) participation, nor do we know about the accuracy of the parents' reports. Other research has found that parents report higher levels of school meal participation than do children (Gordon et all 2007), and parents' reports do not clearly distinguish between breakfasts obtained from the School Breakfast Program versus other food that may be available at the school. Our reports of usual participation are higher than usual participation among all public elementary school students as reported in the SNDA-III (Gordon et al 2007) (40.8 percent versus 31.2 percent), which could reflect our use of parent-reported participation as compared to the SNDA-III use of child-reported participation. Differences could also reflect different sample frames: our sample is limited to 3rd graders, who may or may not participate at rates comparable to all elementary school students. With regard to our breakfast-skipping analysis, we are likewise limited to parents' reports, which may or may not be an accurate reflection of children's behavior. And, we know from past research that analyses of the determinants of breakfast-skipping are sensitive to the specific definition of breakfast that is used (see, e.g., Devaney & Stuart 1998).

Predicted probabilities are based on probit model of marginal food security among children below 185% of poverty line, using data from Early Childhood Longitudinal Survey—Kindergarten Cohort, wave 5, restricted access files (see Table 5). Predictions assume the following characteristics: household is in rural Midwest in county with median rent of $600/month; school has free and reduced price meal certification rate of 25%; student is white and lives with single employed mother who rents home and is in good health with high school education, two children, and annual income of $15,001 -$20,000.

REFERENCES

Bartfeld, J. & Dunifon, R. (2006). "State-Level Predictors of Household Food Security Among Households With Children." *Journal of Policy Analysis and Management, 24(4)*, 921- 942.

Bartfeld, J. & Wang, L. (2006). *Local-level Predictors of Household Food Insecurity*. Final Report for the Institute for Research on Poverty.

Bernell, S., Weber, B. & Edwards, M. (2004). *"Restricted Opportunities, Poor Personal Choices, Failed Policies, Social Decay? What Explains Food Insecurity in Oregon?"* Paper presented at the Association for Public Policy Analysis and Management Annual research conference, Atlanta, GA, October 28-30, 2004.

Bernstein, L. S., McLaughlin, J. E., Crepinsek, M. K. & Daft, L. M. (2004). *Evaluation of the School Breakfast Program Pilot Project. Final Report.* Nutrition Assistance Program.

Report Series No. CN-04-SBP. U.S. Department of Agriculture, Food and Nutrition Service, Office of Analysis, *Nutrition, and Evaluation,* Alexandria, VA.

Bhattacharya, J., Currie, J. & Haider, S. (2004). *Breakfast of Champions? The School Breakfast Program and the Nutrition of Children and Families.* NBER Working Paper 10608.

Devaney, B. & Stuart, E. (1998). "Eating Breakfast: Effects of the School Breakfast Program." *Family Economics and Nutrition Review*, 60-62.

Figlio, D. N., Gundersen, C. & Ziliak, J. P. (2000). "The Food Stamp Program in an Era of Welfare Reform." *American Journal of Agricultural Economics, 83(2)*, 635-658.

Food and Nutrition Service, U.S. Department of Agriculture. (2009). School Breakfast Program Participation and Meals Served._*http://www.fn s.usda.gov/pd/sbsummar.htm*. Accessed June 18.

Food Research and Action Center. (2002). *School Breakfast Scorecard. 2002.*

Washington, D.C.: FRAC.

Food Research and Action Center. (2007). *School Breakfast Scorecard. 2007.* Washington, D.C.: FRAC.

Fox, M. K., Crepinsek, M. K. & Connor, P. (2001). *The Second School Nutrition Dietary Assessment Study (SNDA-II). Final Report.* U.S. Department of Agriculture, Food and Nutrition Service.

Fox, M. K., Hamilton, W. & Lin, B. H. (2004). *Effects of Food Assistance and Nutriton Programs on Nutrition and Health.* Food Assistance and Nutrition Research Report No. FANRR19-4. U.S. Department of Agriculture, Economic Research Service. December.

Gleason, P. M. (1995). "Participation in the National School Lunch Program and the School Breakfast Program." *American Journal of Clinical Nutrition, 61(S)*, 213S-220S.

Gleason, P. M. & Suitor, C. (2001). *Children's Diets in the Mid-1990's: Dietary Intake and Its Relationship with School Meal Participation.* U.S. Department of Agriculture, Food and Nutrition Service.

Gordon, A. & Fox, M. K. (2007). *School Nutrition Dietry Assessment Study—III. Summary of Findings.* Princeton, NJ: Mathematica Policy Research, Inc.

Gordon, A., Fox, M. K., Clark, M., Nogales, R., Elizabeth, C., Gleason, P. & Sarin, A. (2007). *School Nutrition Dietary Assessment Study—III: Volume II: Student Participation and Dietary Intke.* Princeton, NJ: Mathematica Policy Research, Inc.

Haines, J., Neumark-Sztainer, D., Wall, M. & Story, M. (2007). "Personal, Behavioral, and Environmental Risk and Protective Factors for Adolescent Overweight." *Obesity, 15*, 2748-2760.

Jyoti, D. F., Frongillo, E. A. & Jones, S. J. (2005). "Food Insecurity Affects School Children's Academic Performance, Weight Gain, and Social Skills." *Journal of Nutrition, 135*, 283 1- 2839.

Kennedy, E. & Davis, C. (1998). "U.S. Department of Agriculture School Breakfast Program." *American Journal of Clinical Nutrition* 67(Suppl):798S-803 S.

Lent, M. & Emerson, B. (2007). *Preliminary Findings from the 2006-200 7 Universal Free Breakfast Initiative in Milwaukee Public Schools.* Milwaukee, WI: Hunger Task Force of Milwaukee.

McLaughlin, J. E., Bernstein, L. S., Crepinsek, M. K., Daft, L. M., & Murphy, J. M. (2002). *Evaluation of the School Breakfast Program Pilot Project. Findings From the First Year of Implementation.* Nutrition Assistance Report Program Report Series, Report No. RCN-02-SBP. U.S.

Department of Agriculture, Food and Nutrition Service.

National Center for Educational Statistics. (1999). *ECLS-K Base Year Data Files and Electronic Codebook.*

Nord, M. & Romig, K. (2006). "Hunger in the Summer: Seasonal Food Insecurity and the National School Lunch and Summer Food Service Programs." *Journal of Children and Poverty, 12(2)*, 141-158.

Nord, M., Dunifon, R. & Bartfeld, J. (2005). "Measuring Household Food Security in Self- Administered Surveys." Working paper.

Reddan, J., Wahlstrom, K. & Reicks, M. (2002). "Children's Perceived Benefits and Barriers in Relation to Eating Breakfast in Schools With or Without Universal School Breakfast." *Journal of Nutrition Education and Behavior, 34(1)*, 47-52.

Rosales, W. & Janowski, J. (2002). *The State of Breakfast in Wisconsin.* Milwaukee, WI: Hunger Task Force of Milwaukee.

U.S. Department of Agriculture. (2008). *The School Breakfast Program.* U.S. Department of Agriculture, Food and Nutrition Service. http://www.fns.usda.gov/cnd/breakfast/AboutBFast/SBPFactSheet.pdf. Accessed June 18, 2009.

Waehrer, G. (2007). *The School Breakfast Program and Breakfast Consumption.* Final report submitted to the Institute for Research on Poverty.

Wilde, P. (2007). "Measuring the Effect of Food Stamps on Food Insecurity and Hunger: Research and Policy Considerations." *Journal of Nutrition, 137*, 307-3 10.

Winicki, J. & Jemison, K. (2003). "Food Insecurity and Hunger in the Kindergarten Classroom: Its Effect on Learning and Growth." *Contemporary Economic Policy, 21*, 145-157.

Wong, K. & Emerson, B. (2006). *Evaluation of the 2005-2006 Provision 2 Pilot in Milwaukee Public Schools.* Milwaukee: Hunger Task Force of Milwaukee.

Yen, W. T. &rews, M., Chen, Z. & Eastwood, D. B. (2007). "Food Stamp Program Participation and Food Insecurity: An Instrumental Variables Approach." *American Journal of Agricultural Economics, 90(1)*, 117-132.

Ziliak, J. P., Gundersen, C. & Figlio, D. N. (2003). "Food Stamp Caseloads Over the Business Cycle." *Southern Economic Journal, 69(4)*, 903-920.

End Notes

[1] The ECLS-K does not directly ask about skipped meals. It does include information about the number of meals eaten at home and at school, but the information on meals at school is only asked of the subset of respondents who report that the child usually participates in the School Breakfast Program. As such, school breakfasts for occasional participants are not counted, and estimates of breakfast skipping are biased upward.

[2] These are schools for which a non-trivial number of parents reported that their child eats breakfast at school, but the School Breakfast Program is not offered, according to official information. These appear to be schools that offer breakfast or morning snack programs that are not connected to the School Breakfast Program.

[3] We compare self-reported participation rates to official certification rates, rather than official participation rates, as the latter are not available at the school level.

[4] For this as well as the subsequent models, we also experimented with logit models; results are not sensitive to functional form.

[5] Note that, for our original sample of 10350 children, 2050 are missing information from school administrators regarding availability of school breakfast. These children are excluded from the participation analysis.

[6] CPS results are based on analyses conducted by Mark Nord, Economic Research Service, U.S.D.A., August 2008.

In: Meals in School: Issues and Impacts ISBN: 978-1-61209-127-3
Editors: Dayna A. Michalka et al. © 2011 Nova Science Publishers, Inc.

Chapter 2

THE SCHOOL BREAKFAST PROGRAM: PARTICIPATION AND IMPACTS

Judi Bartfeld, Myoung Kim, Jeong Hee Ryu and Hong-Min Ahn

1. WHAT IS THE SCHOOL BREAKFAST PROGRAM?

The School Breakfast Program is a federally assisted meal program operating in public and nonprofit private schools and residential child care institutions. It began as a pilot project in 1966, and was made permanent in 1975. The School Breakfast Program is administered at the Federal level by the Food and Nutrition Service. At the State level, the program is usually administered by State education agencies, which operate the program through agreements with local school food authorities in more than 87,000 schools and institutions.

2. HOW DOES THE SCHOOL BREAKFAST PROGRAM WORK?

The School Breakfast Program operates in the same manner as the National School Lunch Program. Generally, public or nonprofit private schools of high school grade or under and public or nonprofit private residential child care institutions may participate in the School Breakfast Program. School districts and independent schools that choose to take part in the breakfast program receive cash subsidies from the U.S. Department of Agriculture (USDA) for each meal they serve. In return, they must serve breakfasts that meet Federal requirements, and they must offer free or reduced price breakfasts to eligible children.

3. WHAT ARE THE NUTRITIONAL REQUIREMENTS FOR SCHOOL BREAKFASTS?

School breakfasts must meet the applicable recommendations of the Dietary Guidelines for Americans which recommend that no more than 30 percent of an individual's calories come from fat, and less than 10 percent from saturated fat. In addition, breakfasts must provide one-fourth of the Recommended Dietary Allowance for protein, calcium, iron, Vitamin A, Vitamin C and calories. The decisions about what specific food to serve and how they are prepared are made by local school food authorities.

4. HOW DO CHILDREN QUALIFY FOR FREE AND REDUCED PRICE BREAKFASTS?

Any child at a participating school may purchase a meal through the School Breakfast Program. Children from families with incomes at or below 130 percent of the Federal poverty level are eligible for free meals. Those with incomes between 130 percent and 185 percent of the poverty level are eligible for reduced-price meals. (For the period July 1, 2010, through June 30, 2011, 130 percent of the poverty level is $28,665 for a family of four; 185 percent is $40,793.) Children from families over 185 percent of poverty pay full price, though their meals are still subsidized to some extent.

5. HOW MUCH REIMBURSEMENT DO SCHOOLS GET?

Most of the support USDA provides to schools in the School Breakfast Program comes in the form of a cash reimbursement for each breakfast served.

The current (July 1, 2010 through June 30, 2011) basic cash reimbursement rates for non-severe need are:

- Free breakfasts $1.48
- Reduced-price breakfasts $1.18
- Paid breakfasts $0.26

Schools may qualify for higher "severe need" reimbursements if 40% of their lunches are served free or at a reduced price in the second preceding year. Severe need payments are up to 28 cents higher than the normal reimbursements for free and reduced -price breakfasts. About 74 percent of the breakfasts served in the School Breakfast Program receive severe need payments. Higher reimbursement rates are in effect for Alaska and Hawaii.

Schools may charge no more than 30 cents for a reduced-price breakfast. Schools set their own prices for breakfasts served to students who pay the full meal price (paid), though they must operate their meal services as non-profit programs.

For the latest reimbursement rates visit FNS website at
www.fns.usda.gov/cnd/Governance/notices/naps/NAPs.htm

6. WHAT OTHER SUPPORT DO SCHOOLS GET FROM USDA?

Through Team Nutrition, USDA provides schools with technical training and assistance to help school food service staffs prepare healthy meals, and with nutrition education to help children understand the link between diet and health.

7. HOW MANY CHILDREN HAVE BEEN SERVED OVER THE YEARS?

In Fiscal Year 2007, over 10.1 million children participated every day. That number grew to over 11.1 million in Fiscal Year 2009. Of those, 9.1 million received their meals free or at a reduced-price.

Participation has slowly but steadily grown over the years: 1970: 0.5 million children; 1975: 1.8 million children; 1980: 3.6 million children; 1985:

3.4 million children; 1990: 4.0 million children; 1995: 6.3 million children; 2000: 7.5 million children.

8. HOW MUCH DOES THE PROGRAM COST?

For Fiscal Year 2009, the School Breakfast Program cost $2.9 billion, up from $1.9 billion in Fiscal Year 2005. The cost in previous years was in 1970, $ 10.8 million; in 1980, $287.8 million; in 1990, $ 599.1 million; and in 2000, $1.39 billion.

For more information:

For information on the operation of the School Breakfast Program and all the Child Nutrition Programs, contact the State agency in your state that is responsible for the administration of the programs. A listing of all our State agencies may be found on our web site at www.fns.usda.gov/cnd, select "Contact Us" then select "Child Nutrition Programs."

You may also contact us through the Office of Public Affairs (CGA) at 703 -305-2281, or by mail at 3101 Park Center Drive, Room 914, Alexandria, Virginia 22302.

September 2010

In: Meals in School: Issues and Impacts   ISBN: 978-1-61209-127-3
Editors: Dayna A. Michalka et al.   © 2011 Nova Science Publishers, Inc.

Chapter 3

MEETING TOTAL FAT REQUIREMENTS FOR SCHOOL LUNCHES: INFLUENCE OF SCHOOL POLICIES AND CHARACTERISTICS

Constance Newman, Joanne Guthrie, Lisa Mancino,
Katherine Ralston and Melissa Musiker

ABSTRACT

Concerns about child obesity have raised questions about the quality of meals served in the National School Lunch Program. Local, State, and Federal policymakers responded to these concerns beginning in the mid-1990s by instituting a range of policies and standards to improve the quality of U.S. Department of Agriculture-subsidized meals. Schools have been successful in meeting USDA nutrient standards except those for total fat and saturated fat. This chapter uses school-level data from the School Nutrition Dietary Assessment-III to calculate statistical differences between the fat content of NSLP lunches served by schools with different policies (e.g., menu planning) and characteristics like region and size. Positive associations are found between a meal's fat content and the presence of a la carte foods and vending machines, which are thought to indirectly affect the nutrient content of USDA-subsidized meals.

Keywords: National School Lunch Program (NSLP), obesity, nutrition

SUMMARY

Concerns about child obesity have raised questions about the quality of meals served in the National School Lunch Program (NSLP). Local, State, and Federal policymakers responded to these concerns beginning in the mid-1990s by instituting a range of policies and standards to improve the quality of USDA-subsidized meals. While most of USDA's nutrition standards have been met by schools, total fat and saturated fat as a percent of calories is an ongoing challenge.

What Is the Issue?

The School Nutrition Dietary Assessment-III, conducted by USDA's Food and Nutrition Service, recently found that while most schools meet requirements for vitamins, protein, calcium, and iron, only one in five schools served lunches that met the standard for total fat, set at 30 percent of calories or less. This chapter compares the characteristics and food policies of schools serving lunches that met total fat requirements to those serving lunches with fat content that was either 30-35 percent of calories (middle category) or over 35 percent (high). Identifying the food practices and policies of conforming versus nonconforming schools may help to identify effective strategies for improving the nutritional quality of USDA school meals.

What Did the Study Find?

The fat content of school lunches was statistically correlated with many school policies and characteristics in the spring of 2005. Some policies and practices, such as whether french fries are regularly served, can directly affect the nutritional content of USDA lunches. Other policies, such as a school's allowance of "competitive" foods or foods that bypass nutritional standards, can indirectly affect the content of USDA lunches by offering choices that appeal to students' taste preferences. Among the policies or practices that directly affect the fat content of USDA lunches:

- *Promotion of fresh fruits and vegetables/local foods*. Participation in at least one program that promotes the purchase of locally grown food or fresh fruit and vegetables was significantly higher in elementary and middle/high schools that serve lunches in the lowest fat category, below 30 percent of calories.

- *French fries or dessert.* The provision of french fries or dessert as a part of the USDA lunch was significantly higher among middle/high schools in the highest fat category.

- *Low-fat milk only.* Providing lowfat milk as the only milk choice was significantly higher in the lowest fat category for both elementary and middle/high schools.

- *Meal planning method.* Historically, schools have used a food-based ("traditional") method for planning menus where each meal must consist of certain food types such as a meat, vegetable, starch, etc. In recent years, some schools have adopted a nutrient-based method where lunches are planned according to the nutrient content of food items, or they use a mix of methods called the "enhanced traditional" method. The traditional meal planning method was used significantly more by schools in the highest fat category for both elementary and middle/high schools, whereas the enhanced traditional method was used more in the lowest fat category for middle/high schools.

Other policies may affect lunch quality since they enable students to choose alternative foods. For example, the availability of a la carte foods in elementary schools was significantly higher in the middle category of fat content than in the lowest category; no relationship across fat categories was found for middle/high schools. And the presence of vending machines was significantly higher among middle/high schools in the highest fat category.

Although school characteristics (rural vs. urban, region, size) are not subject to policy change, they may be useful for targeting lunch improvement efforts. For both elementary and middle/high schools, urban schools were more highly represented in the lowest fat category, and rural schools were more predominant in the highest fat category. Elementary and middle/high schools in the Southeast were more predominant in the two higher fat categories than in the lowest category, whereas Southwest schools were more predominant in the two lower fat categories. Elementary schools in the West were more pre-dominant in the lowest fat category than in the two higher fat categories.

How Was the Study Conducted?

We used nationally representative school-level data from the School Nutrition Dietary Assessment-III to calculate the statistical effect of school policies and characteristics on the fat content of NSLP lunches served by 397 schools. Schools were divided into three categories based on the average fat content of reimbursable school lunches served and chosen by students over a week. The fat content categories were (1) no more than 30 percent of calories from fat, (2) 30 to 35 percent of calories from fat, and (3) more than 35 percent of calories from fat. We compared the policies, practices, and characteristics of schools within each fat category to those in the other two fat categories. Using a student's t-test and school-level sample weights, we indicate mean differences between subgroups that vary with a 90-percent level of significance or above. This threshold was chosen because of small sample size, especially among specific fat content subcategories.

INTRODUCTION

Every weekday, schools around the country strive to provide students with a healthy lunch. To qualify for Federal subsidies under the National School Lunch Program (NSLP), school meals must meet USDA nutrition requirements. At the same time, to fulfill the nutrition goals of the program and maintain the financial viability of the program, these meals must be sufficiently appealing for students to select them.

Since the development of new school meal nutrition standards in the mid-1990s, USDA has emphasized lowering the fat content of school meals. Yet meeting standards for fat and saturated fat remains a problem. A recent study sponsored by USDA's Food and Nutrition Service, School Nutrition Dietary Assessment-III (SNDA-III), found that most schools meet the requirements for vitamins, protein, calcium, and iron. However, few schools meet the total fat and saturated fat requirements (Figure 1).[1] One in five schools served lunches that met the standard for total fat and almost a third met the standard for saturated fat in 2005.

What do we know about the schools that did meet or failed to meet these requirements? This chapter uses SNDA-III data to compare the food policies, practices, and characteristics of schools that met total fat requirements to those that did not. Identifying such correlations may help to devise strategies for improving the nutritional quality of USDA school meals.

We use SNDA-III school-level data collected from 397 schools in the spring of 2005. Schools fall into one of three categories based on the average fat content of reimbursable school lunches served and chosen by students over a week (henceforth referred to as "served"). An analysis of lunches offered would not fully account for the fact that students usually have some choices, such as the choice between higher or lower fat milk, so this analysis is based on the lunches chosen by students. This measure provides an estimate that considers both the nutritional quality of the items offered by schools and their acceptability to students.[2]

The fat content categories are (1) no more than 30 percent of calories from fat, (2) 30 to 35 percent of calories from fat, and (3) more than 35 percent of calories from fat. Current NSLP total fat standards are based on the *Dietary Guideline for Americans* released in 2000, which recommend keeping fat intake below 30 percent of calories. The 2005 *Dietary Guideline for Americans* relaxed the standard for fat intake to between 25 and 35 percent of calories. Assuming that the NSLP standards will be updated to refl ect the change, we identify schools that would meet a requirement of 35 percent but not 30 percent total fat. We report nationally representative results using the school-level sample weights.

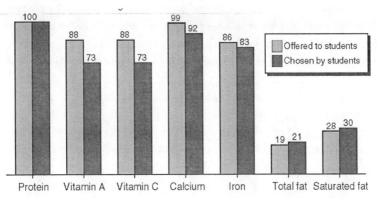

Source: USDA, Food and Nutrition Service. School Nutrition Dietary Assessment-III, Menu Survey, Nutrition Assistance Program Report Series, November 2007.

Figure 1. Most schools meet USDA nutrition standards for National School Lunch Program lunches except for total fat and saturated fat, 2005 Percent of schools meeting USDA standards

Table 1. School Lunch Fat Categories by School Type, 2005

Sample shares	Total fat < 30% (kcals)	Total fat 30-35% (kcals)	Total fat > 35% (kcals)
Unweighted sample N = 397	n = 76	n = 172	n = 149
	Percent		
Weighted sample 100	21	40	39
School type			
• Elementary school (63%) 100	26*	43	31*
• Middle/high school (37%) 100	12*	36	52*

* Significant difference between elementary and middle/high schools at the 99% level.
Source: USDA, Economic Research Service, based on calculations from SNDA III.

This work complements research that analyzes the effect of school environments on children's dietary outcomes (Briefel et al., 2009) and children's obesity (Fox et al., 2009) and research that summarizes the characteristics of school environments (Finkelstein et al., 2008; GAO, 2005). Clark and Fox (2009) find that the total fat intake over 24 hours was not higher among NSLP participants than nonparticipants, but that for all children, 24-hour total fat intake exceeded 2005 Dietary Guidelines.

Almost two-thirds of the schools in the weighted sample are elementary schools (63 percent), while 37 percent are middle schools and high schools combined (table 1). Elementary schools were more likely to comply with fat requirements than were middle and high schools, and the differences are statistically significant, meaning they are unlikely to be due to chance. Among elementary schools, 26 percent served lunches that met the requirement (less than 30 percent fat), 43 percent served lunches in the middle category of fat content (between 30 and 35 percent fat), and 31 percent served lunches in the highest fat content category (over 35 percent fat). Among middle/high schools, 12 percent served lunches with the lowest fat content, 36 percent served lunches in the middle category of fat content, and 52 percent served lunches in the highest fat content category.

These results are consistent with other research findings that older students face a less healthy school food environment (Finkelstein et al., 2008; Briefel et al., 2009). Given these large differences and the fact that school food envi-ronments differ greatly by school type, we examine elementary and middle/ high schools separately.

**Table 2. Percent Energy from Total Fat by Fat
Category and School Type, 2005**

		Mean	Median	Minimum	Maximum
Elementary	Total fat < 30% (kcals)	28.1	28.0	22.6	29.9
	Total fat 30-35% (kcals)	32.6	32.6	30.3	35.0
	Total fat > 35% (kcals)	37.3	36.7	35.0	43.8
Middle/High	Total fat < 30% (kcals)	28.2	28.5	23.1	29.9
	Total fat 30-35% (kcals)	32.9	33.1	30.0	34.9
	Total fat > 35% (kcals)	39.0	37.8	35.0	69.5

Table 2 shows the distribution (mean, median, range) of our main variable of interest—the percent of calories from total fat in served meals—within each of the three fat categories. The grouping of the variable helps to identify thresholds that are relevant to USDA requirements, but it is also important to ensure that the underlying distributions of each group can be credibly differentiated. The means refl ect a spread of 28 to 37 percent of calories from fat across the three categories for elementary schools and a spread of 28 to 39 percent of calories from fat for middle and high schools.

SCHOOL FOOD POLICIES AND ENVIRONMENTS

Many school food policies are determined at the State and local levels. In recent years, concerns about obesity and school nutrition have led to a variety of new policies. For example, in 2004 Congress required NSLP-participating schools to establish "Local Wellness Policies," which set locally defined nutrition and physical activity goals for improving student health. Such policies have included the introduction of new nutrition education activities or the removal of access to less healthy foods (such as those found in vending machines). And district- or school-level policy changes have occurred independently in schools where local wellness policies may not be fully established. Some States have also entered the child nutrition policy arena by establishing laws for food purchases by school food managers and the availability of competitive foods (i.e., foods that are not served as part of the reimbursable lunch).

We examine policies and practices that can directly affect USDA lunches, such as whether french fries are ever served, and others that can indirectly affect USDA lunches, such as the presence of competitive foods. We divide school policies, whether indirect or direct, into four general types:

- **Competitive food policies** include the presence of vending machines and/or a la carte foods, which may indirectly affect the fat content of USDA lunches by providing students with alternative lunches.
- **Nutrition and purchasing policies**, such as whether the school has a local wellness policy, nutrition education, or nutrient-related food purchasing, may directly or indirectly affect the fat content of USDA lunches.
- **Participation in special programs**, such as programs that promote fresh fruit and vegetables or locally produced foods, is thought to directly affect the fat content of USDA lunches.
- **Menu and food preparation characteristics**, such as whether the menus are planned at the district level or whether food is prepared onsite, directly affect the fat content of the USDA lunch.

We examine how each type of policy may be linked to lunch fat content and the findings for both elementary and middle/high schools. All differences across lunch fat categories are statistically significant differences, unless otherwise noted. We use a significance level of 90 percent (rather than 95 percent) because of the relatively small sample size.

Information about school-level policies was obtained from different sources: the school principal, the school foodservice manager, or a school food authority/SFA (or district) representative. In the few cases where answers differed among sources, we use data developed by the researchers who conducted the survey. They identified the best sources by comparing responses to checklist surveys that they conducted on school grounds.

Presence of Competitive Foods

The presence of competitive foods in schools has recently come under scrutiny amid concern about children's diets. Of special concern are vending machines and a la carte foods, offered alongside NSLP lunches, that are low-nutrition and energy-dense.[3] Competitive foods are usually offered as a way to raise revenue for SFAs who operate as nonprofit providers of the NSLP meals. Most SFAs operate on a break-even basis, and they say that competitive food sales are necessary to cover their costs. School principals, athletic departments, and clubs may also decide to raise revenue through vending machines, school stores, or bake sales.

Competitive foods are so named because they are widely thought to deter NSLP participation by providing an alternative, usually less healthy, lunch for students to choose. To attract students to the NSLP lunch, schools may provide lunches with a higher fat content than would be offered if competitive foods were not available. Also, students may choose reimbursable lunch items with higher fat content than they would choose if competitive foods were not available. The availability of snacks or sweets at school through small stores or bake sale-type fundraising activities has raised similar concerns that the NSLP lunch must "compete" with these foods to be attractive to students. Access to soft drinks and other sweetened beverages is also under scrutiny in schools because of their possible links to obesity. The existence of "pouring contracts," where a school gives exclusive sales rights to a beverage company, is thought to be associated with greater access to sweetened beverages. That access may also work against the attractiveness of a lower-fat NSLP lunch. To combat this, some schools have restrictions on food and beverage availability.

To test the relationship between a lunch's fat content and access to competitive food, we examine the correlations between the fat content of lunches served and the availability of: a la carte food of any kind; a la carte food that is low- nutrition, energy-dense; vending machines; vending machines in the foodservice area; pouring contracts; snack bars; school stores; fundraising activities that include sweets or snacks; and food/beverage restrictions (table 3). Large differences in competitive food policy are apparent between elementary and middle/high schools. For example, fewer than 1 in 5 elementary schools have vending machines, whereas 9 out of 10 middle and high schools do. And some policies are adopted much more than others. For example, 78 percent of elementary schools serve a la carte food, while only 9 percent of them have a snack bar or school store.

Elementary Schools

The share of elementary schools selling a la carte food is significantly lower for schools in the lowest fat category (65 percent) than in the middle category (90 percent). Also the share of schools selling low-nutrition, energy-dense foods a la carte was significantly lower in the lowest fat category (23 percent) than in the middle category (50 percent).

Other significant differences were found for the presence of a school store and fundraising activities. Schools with lunches in the lowest fat category had the lowest share of school stores or snack bars (though not significantly lower than schools in the highest fat category). Schools in the middle fat category had the highest share of fundraising activities that sell sweets or snacks (though not significantly higher than schools in the highest fat category).

We found no significant differences among fat categories by vending machine policy. However, this is likely due to small sample size. Only 16 percent of elementary schools had vending machines present in schools.

Middle and High Schools

Among middle and high schools, schools in the highest fat category were significantly more likely to have vending machines (96 percent) than were schools in the other two categories (table 3). Contrary to expectations, however, schools in the highest fat category were significantly less likely to have low-nutrition, energy-dense food in the a la carte line (43 percent) than schools in either of the other two categories (77 percent low and 62 percent middle). Surprisingly, schools did not differ much in fat content by the other competitive food policies, such as pouring rights or presence of vending in the foodservice area.

Nutrition and Purchasing Policies

With increasing interest in school nutrition, schools have instituted various types of nutrition promotion policies that may be correlated with the provision and acceptance of lower fat lunches. We compare lunch fat content across schools with different nutrition policies, such as whether they have nutrient requirements for food purchases, schoolwide wellness policies,[4] nutrition education, and/or nutrition and health advisory councils. Another variable that we consider is whether schools use "Child Nutrition (CN) label foods," a class of foods—mainly pre-prepared foods such as pizzas, burritos, etc.—that are specially marketed for USDA school meals and carry a label indicating how they meet the traditional food group requirements of a meal (how much of the required serving of meat, grain, etc.). CN labels, unlike the standard nutrition labels found on foods in supermarkets, do not contain information on fat or saturated fat content.

-- Table 3. Presence of Competitive Foods by Fat Category and School Type, 2005

	Sample share or mean	Total fat < 30% (kcals)	Total fat 30-35% (kcals)	Total fat > 35% (kcals)
Elementary schools – unweighted sample	N = 144	n = 42	n = 69	n = 33
		Percent		
A la carte food sold	78	65[12]	90[12]	72
Low-nutrition, energy-dense food sold a la carte (if any sold)	40	23[12]	50[12]	41
Vending machines present	16	11	18	19
Vending machines in foodservice area (if vending present)	11	10	7	18
Pouring contracts	46	51	47	39
School store or snack bar sells snacks	9	3[12]	11[12]	9
Fundraising activities that sell sweets or snacks	36	31	46[23]	25[23]
Restrictions on type of food or snacks sold	39	43	42	33
Restrictions on type of sweet beverages sold	49	52	54	41
Middle and high schools - unweighted sample	N = 253	n = 34	n = 103	n = 116
		Percent		
A la carte food sold	82	81	89	77
Low-nutrition, energy-dense food sold a la carte (if any sold)	55	77[13]	62[23]	43[13,23]
Vending machines present	88	67[13]	84[23]	96[13,23]
Vending machines in foodservice area (if vending present)	44	41	41	46
Pouring contracts	71	69	68	74
School store or snack bar sells snacks	21	31	20	19
Fundraising activities that sell sweets or snacks	53	57	45	59
Restrictions or ban on type of food or snacks sold	37	36	41	34
Restrictions or ban on type of sweet beverages sold	50	57	52	46

[12] Significant difference between category 1 and 2 at the 90% level.

[23] Significant difference between category 2 and 3 at the 90% level.

[13] Significant difference between category 1 and 3 at the 90% level.

Source: USDA, Economic Research Service, based on calculations from SNDA III.

Table 4. Nutrition and purchasing policies by fat category and school type, 2005

	Sample share or mean	Total fat < 30% (kcals) (1)	Total fat 30-35% (kcals) (2)	Total fat > 35% (kcals) (3)
Elementary schools – unweighted sample	N = 144	n = 42	n = 69	n = 33
		Percent		
School has a wellness policy	48	44	54	37
School has nutrition education at every grade	80	78	76	87
School has a nutrition or health advisory council	18	15	19	23
School routinely makes nutrition info available to parents	60	61	67	53
District purchases are based on nutrient requirements	52	48	61^{23}	38^{23}
District requires Child Nutrition* label for some or all foods	63	49^{12}	71^{12}	69
Some foods offered from chain restaurants	30	39	30	23
Middle and high schools - unweighted sample	N = 253	n = 34	n = 103	n = 116
		Percent		
School has a wellness policy	37	46	38	34
School has nutrition education at every grade	53	57	50	46
School has a nutrition or health advisory council	21	25	26	27
School routinely makes nutrition info available to parents	58	75^{12}	54^{12}	58
District purchases are based on nutrient requirements	56	55	65	53
District requires CN* label for some or all foods	64	67	71	60
Some or all foods offered from chain restaurants	27	39	26	21

* CN = Child Nutrition.

[12] Significant difference between category 1 and 2 at the 90% level. 23 Significant difference between category 2 and 3 at the 90% level.

[13] Significant difference between category 1 and 3 at the 90% level.

Source: USDA, Economic Research Service, based on calculations from SNDA III.

Elementary Schools

Elementary schools in the middle fat category were significantly more likely to have district purchases based on nutrition requirements than were schools in the highest fat category (table 4), and were significantly more likely to be in districts requiring CN labels than schools in the lowest fat category. Other nutrition-related policies did not differ significantly across the lunch fat categories, and in many cases, the differences were the opposite of those expected. For example, schools with nutrition education and a nutrition advisory council were not significantly more likely to be in the lowest fat category. And schools serving foods from chain restaurants were not more likely to be in the highest fat category.

Middle and High Schools

The only statistically significant nutrition and purchasing policy difference across lunch fat categories was whether schools make nutrition information available to parents on a routine basis, such as sending home daily menus (table 4). Schools in the lowest fat category were significantly more likely to have this policy (75 percent) than schools in the middle category (54 percent).

Participation in Special Fruit and Vegetable Purchasing Programs

We examine differences in lunch fat content based on schools' participation in programs designed to increase the availability of fresh food, and in particular, fresh fruit and vegetables. These policies include whether the school district participated in a State or local farm-to-school program,[5] whether the district participated in the U.S. Department of Defense's Fresh Fruit and Vegetable Program,[6] and whether the State or district has regulations that require purchase of locally produced foods or fresh produce.

Elementary Schools

Schools that participated in at least one of the special programs (table 5) were significantly more likely to be in the lowest fat category (62 percent) and middle category (63 percent) than in the highest fat category (37 percent). Across individual programs, there were few significant differences, but in three out of four programs, the schools in the middle fat category were the most highly represented.

Middle and High Schools

Similar to the elementary school results, participation in at least one special program was significantly higher for middle/high schools in the lowest and middle fat categories (68 and 61 percent, respectively) than in the highest fat category (43 percent) (table 5).

Table 5. Participation in special programs by fat category and school type, 2005

	Sample share or mean	Total fat < 30% (kcals) (1)	Total fat 30-35% (kcals) (2)	Total fat > 35% (kcals) (3)
Elementary schools – Unweighted sample	N = 144	n = 42	n = 69	n = 33
		Percent		
District participates in, or has, any of the programs below	58	62[13]	63[23]	37[12,23]
District has guidelines for buying locally grown	17	28	11	13
District has guidelines for buying fresh produce	11	10	12	10
District buys from Dept. of Defense Fresh program	39	38	52[23]	21[23]
District participates in State farm-to-school program	14	15	16	9
Middle and high schools - Unweighted sample	N = 253	n = 34	n = 103	n = 116
		Percent		
District participates in, or has, any of the programs below	53	68[13]	61[23]	43[13,23]
District has guidelines for buying locally grown	15	21	20	10
District has guidelines for buying fresh produce	8	3[12]	13[12]	6
District buys from Dept. of Defense Fresh program	33	41	33	31
District participates in State farm-to-school program	15	16	16	14

[12] Significant difference between category 1 and 2 at the 90% level.
[23] Significant difference between category 2 and 3 at the 90% level.
[13] Significant difference between category 1 and 3 at the 90% level.
Source: USDA, Economic Research Service, based on calculations from SNDA III.

Menu and Food Preparation Characteristics

Menu and food preparation characteristics include the planning of lunches, the features of lunches (such as whether french fries are served), the average total calorie content, and the share of calories from sources other than fat. In planning meals, some schools have moved from the traditional "food-based" method (where each meal must consist of certain food item types—meat, vegetable, starch, etc.) to a nutrient-based method where meals are planned according to the nutrient content of food items. In theory, this latter method may be a more precise way to meet nutrient requirements, but it also requires more time and sophistication. Less than a third of schools used the nutrient-based method in school year 2004-05. Some schools (22 percent) had opted for the intermediary option of "enhanced" traditional meal planning, which is the food-based method with more fruits, vegetables, grains, and breads.

We hypothesize that schools that have taken specific measures such as not serving either whole or 2-percent milk, not serving french fries, or serving fresh produce daily will be better able to reduce the fat content of their lunches. However, since school lunches are encouraged to provide one-third of students' total daily calories, school lunch providers may add ingredients that are low in fat but still calorie dense, such as simple carbohydrates and added sugars, for which there are currently no specific guidelines.

We also check for correlations between fat content of lunches and various food preparation policies, such as whether the kitchen uses fully plated lunches from offsite. The offsite preparation of food and the use of processed foods are thought to produce higher fat meals (Miller, 2009).

Elementary Schools

In terms of menu planning methods, there were large and significant differences across elementary schools (table 6). Elementary schools in the lowest fat category had a significantly lower share of traditional menu planning (32 percent) than did schools in the highest fat category (67 percent). This is some evidence in favor of nutrient-based planning. Schools in the middle fat category were significantly more likely to have menus planned at the district level (58 percent) than were schools in the highest fat category (35 percent). Limiting milk offerings to low-fat only was the only other menu variable that showed significant differences among fat categories. Elementary schools in the lowest fat category were significantly more likely to serve only low-fat milk (56 percent) than schools in either of the two other categories.

Table 6. Menu and food preparation characteristics by fat category and school type, 2005

	Sample share or mean	Total fat < 30% (kcals) (1)	Total fat 30-35% (kcals) (2)	Total fat > 35% (kcals) (3)
Elementary schools – unweighted sample	N = 144	n = 42	n = 69	n = 33
		Percent		
Type of menu planning				
• Nutrient based	30	39	33	19
• Enhanced	21	29	20	15
• Traditional	49	32[13]	47	67[13]
Menus planned at district-level	55	56	58[23]	35[23]
Menus planned by foodservice management company	9	3	7	15
Fries are offered 1 or more days per week	71	73	67	67
Dessert is offered 1 or more days per week	73	69	80	59
Fresh fruit and vegetables are offered daily	50	39	46	60
Whole milk and 2% milk are not offered	31	56[12,13]	30[12]	20[13]
Mean total calories	676	660[13]	658[23]	714[13,23]
Mean share of calories from protein	16.6	17.3[12,23]	16.8[12,23]	15.9[13,23]
Mean share of calories from carbohydrates	52.0	56.4[12,23]	52.1[12,23]	48.3[13,23]
Mean share of calories from added sugars*	26.7	29.6[12,23]	26.7[12,23]	24.3[13,23]
Which of the following describes your kitchen?				
• Onsite, meals prepared for this site only	67	60	69	70
• Base kitchen, meals prepared for many schools	8	9	7	9
• Receiving kitchen, meals prepared offsite	25	31	24	20
Receive fully plated meals from offsite	9	7	12	6
Middle and high schools - unweighted sample	N = 253	n = 34	n = 103	n = 116
		Percent		
Type of menu planning				
• Nutrient based	28	36	22	31
• Enhanced	22	40[13]	24	16[13]
• Traditional	50	24[12,13]	54[12]	53[13]
Menus planned at district-level	46	44	48	46

Table 6. (Continued)

	Sample share or mean	Total fat < 30% (kcals) (1)	Total fat 30-35% (kcals) (2)	Total fat > 35% (kcals) (3)
Menus planned by food service management company	7	17	9	4
Fries are offered 1 or more days per week	83	$62^{12,13}$	83^{12}	86^{13}
Dessert is offered 1 or more days per week	77	64^{13}	69^{23}	$84^{23,13}$
Fresh fruit and vegetables are offered daily	56	48	52	60
Whole milk and 2% milk are not offered	34	$69^{12,13}$	29^{12}	28^{13}
Mean total calories	765	688^{13}	719^{23}	$814^{13,23}$
Mean share of calories from protein	15.8	16.6^{13}	16.5^{23}	$15.1^{13,23}$
Mean share of calories from carbohydrates	50.2	$57.0^{12,23}$	$52.0^{12,23}$	$47.3^{13,23}$
Mean share of calories from added sugars*	23.7	$30.1^{12,23}$	$24.7^{12,23}$	$21.6^{13,23}$
Which of the following describes your kitchen?				
• Onsite, meals prepared for this site only	77	57^{13}	70^{23}	$87^{13,23}$
• Base kitchen, meals prepared for many schools	15	13	22	11
• Receiving kitchen, meals prepared offsite	8	$30^{12,13}$	$8^{12,13}$	$3^{12,13}$
Receive fully plated meals from offsite	3	5	3	2

* Percent of energy from sugar was calculated by the authors, using variables from SNDA as:

Percent Energy from Sugar =100* (4*Total Sugar)/Total Energy

[12] Significant difference between category 1 and 2 at the 90% level.

[23] Significant difference between category 2 and 3 at the 90% level.

[13] Significant difference between category 1 and 3 at the 90% level.

Source: SDA, Economic Research Service, based on calculations from SNDA III.

Elementary schools that served higher fat lunches served more caloric lunches, on average, as well. This was not surprising as fat has more calories per gram than either carbohydrates or protein. We also found that protein and carbohydrate content varied significantly across the three fat catego-ries. Because a calorie is made of fat, protein, or carbohydrate, a lower fat lunch will also contain more protein, carbohydrates or both. However, across fat categories, the variation in carbohydrates was more pronounced than the variation in protein across fat categories. Also, more than half of carbohydrates came from sugars, suggesting schools may find it easier to lower fat (and maintain total calories) by adding more sugar than by adding more complex carbohydrates such as vegetables and whole grains. This also illuminates a possible unintended consequence of focusing guidelines too narrowly on fat content alone.

Middle and High Schools

Menu planning and food preparation policies seem to differ more at the middle and high school level (table 6). As with elementary schools, schools in the lowest fat category were significantly less likely to use traditional menu planning (24 percent) than were schools in the other two categories (53-54 percent), and they were significantly more likely to use enhanced menu planning (40 percent) than were schools in the highest fat category (16 percent). The offering of french fries at least once during the week observed was significantly less likely in the lowest fat category (62 percent) than in the other two categories (83-86 percent), and the offering of dessert at least once a week was signifi- cantly lower in the lowest fat category (64 percent) and the middle category (69 percent) than in the highest fat category (84 percent). Offering only lowfat milk was also significantly more likely in schools in the lowest fat category (69 percent) than in the other two categories (28-29 percent).

As with elementary schools, lower fat lunches in middle and high schools contained significantly more protein and carbohydrates (table 6). While the protein content of middle/high school lunches varied less compared to elementary school lunches, the variation in carbohydrates and sugars was more pronounced. As middle and high school students have more freedom to choose (and higher caloric requirements), school cafeteria managers may find it especially difficult to abide by fat recommendations, and thus add fl avor and calories by adding sugars.

Surprisingly, middle and high schools in the lowest fat category were sig- nificantly less likely to cook lunches onsite and significantly more likely to receive lunches prepared elsewhere. Fifty-seven percent of schools in the lowest fat category had lunches prepared onsite for their site only, versus 70 and 87 percent of the middle and highest fat category schools. Three out of 10 schools in the lowest fat category received lunches prepared offsite, while fewer than 1 in 10 schools in the middle and highest fat categories did so.

SCHOOL CHARACTERISTICS

Identifying characteristics associated with the likelihood of serving lunches that meet fat standards can help to target fat-reduction strategies to the schools most likely to benefit from them. Some differences may refl ect regional and cultural food preferences. Other differences—such as the share of students certified to receive a free or a reduced-price lunch or child poverty rates—may suggest the role of economic factors.

Urbanicity

With 46 percent of the lowest fat lunches served in an urban area, urban elementary schools were statistically more highly represented in the lowest fat category (table 7). And with 73 percent of the highest fat lunches, rural elementary schools ("not near a city") were most highly represented in the highest fat category. Similar to elementary schools, urban middle and high schools were significantly more likely to serve lunches in the lowest or middle fat category than in the highest fat category.

Regions

Some regional differences were also statistically significant across elementary schools. Elementary schools in the Southeast were more likely to serve lunches in either the middle or highest fat category than in the lowest fat category. Elementary schools in the West were more likely to serve lunches in the lowest fat category than in the middle or highest fat category. Mid-Atlantic schools were more likely to serve lunches in the middle category than to serve lunches in the lowest fat category (table 7).

Regional differences were found to be significant for middle and high schools in the Southwest, Mountain, and Southeast (table 7). As with elementary schools, middle/high schools in the Southeast were significantly more likely to be in the middle and highest fat categories than in the lowest fat category. The Southwest also had a relatively high share of schools in the middle fat category, which was significantly different from its share in the highest fat category. Middle/high schools in the Mountain region had high shares in both the lowest and the highest fat categories, and both were significantly different from the Mountain's share in the middle fat category.

Table 7. School characteristics by fat category and school type, 2005

	Sample share or mean	Total fat < 30% (kcals) (1)	Total fat 30-35% (kcals) (2)	Total fat > 35% (kcals) (3)
Elementary schools – Unweighted sample	N = 144	n = 42	n = 69	n = 33
		Percent		
Urbanicity:				
In a city	34	46[13]	41[23]	10[13,23]
Suburb of a city	20	14	26	17
Not near a city	46	40[13]	33[23]	73[13,23]
Region:				
Mid-Atlantic	11	2[12]	17[12]	10
Midwest	19	20	23	14
Mountain	13	16	8	17
Northeast	11	11	7	16
Southeast	18	6[12,13]	24[12]	21[13]
Southwest	16	22	12	14
West	12	23[12, 13]	9[12]	8[13]
School size:				
< 400	35	36	25[23]	48[23]
400-500	23	13[12]	29[12]	22
500-725	31	37	31	25
725-1,000	8	12[13]	10[23]	3[13,23]
> 1,000	3	2	5	2
Percent of free or reduced-price students	47	48	49	42
District child poverty rate:				
< 20 percent	62	66	58	63
20-30 percent	31	24	34	33
> 30 percent	7	10	8	4
Middle and high schools – Unweighted sample	N = 253	n = 34	n = 102	n = 115
		Percent		
Urbanicity:				
In a city	29	45[13]	37[23]	18[13,23]
Suburb of a city	18	15	17	21
Not near a city	53	40	46	61
Region:				
Mid-Atlantic	9	9	8	10

Table 7. (Continued)

	Sample share or mean	Total fat < 30% (kcals) (1)	Total fat 30-35% (kcals) (2)	Total fat > 35% (kcals) (3)
Midwest	17	17	23	13
Mountain	19	22^{12}	$2^{12,23}$	31^{23}
Northeast	8	9	8	8
Southeast	19	$2^{12,13}$	26^{12}	19^{13}
Southwest	14	27	18^{23}	9^{23}
West	12	14	15	10
School size:				
< 400	28	20	25	33
400-500	12	18	14	9
500-725	21	19	17	23
725-1,000	19	23	26^{23}	13^{23}
> 1,000	20	20	18	22
Percent of free or reduced-price students	42	40	46	40
District child poverty rate:				
< 20 percent	62	57	63	63
20-30 percent	31	33	32	30
> 30 eprcent	6	10	5	7

[12] Significant difference between category 1 and 2 at the 90% level. 23 Significant difference between category 2 and 3 at the 90% level.

[13] Significant difference between category 1 and 3 at the 90% level.

Source: SDA, Economic Research Service, based oncalculations from SNDA III.

School Size

The smallest elementary schools (fewer than 400 students) were significantly more likely to serve lunches in the highest (than the middle) fat category, while the next size schools, with 400-500 students, were most likely to serve lunches in the middle fat category (table 7). The only other significant differences by size were among schools with 725 to 1,000 students: they were more likely to serve lunches in the lowest or middle categories than in the highest fat category.

School size differences were not as significant for middle and high schools as they were for elementary schools. The only differences were among schools with 725 to 1,000 students: they were significantly more likely to serve lunches in the middle fat category than in the highest fat category.

Economic Characteristics

We found no statistically significant differences between fat content of school lunches and the two economic characteristics variables: the average share of students receiving free/reduced-price meals and the district's child poverty rate. The lack of statistical differences among these variables may be partially attributed to the small sample size that this survey provides.

CONCLUSION

Our findings show that the average fat content of lunches served in schools does differ across various school policies and characteristics. The presence of a la carte foods and vending machines seems to indirectly affect the fat content of USDA lunches, though there was no evidence of a relationship between lunch fat content and other competitive food policies such as pouring rights, food and beverage restrictions, and other sources of snacks.

Nutrition and food-purchasing policies—such as wellness policies, nutrition and health councils, and nutrition education—did not correlate with the fat content in school lunches. Many lunch planning characteristics—such as menu planning method; the offering of french fries, desserts, or fruits/vegetables; and offering only low-fat milk—were significant, especially for high schools.

As a caveat to all of the findings, we may be understating the statistical significance of the associations due to the relatively small sample size. However, these data are unique in providing very high-quality nutrition information as well as good detail on school characteristics, and they document many relevant correlations between school characteristics, policies, and the fat content of school lunches. A la carte provision of foods, vending machines, and traditional meal planning are all significantly associated with higher fat lunches. And elementary or middle/high schools with the lowest fat lunches are more likely to participate in at least one program that promotes school purchases of fresh fruits and vegetables or locally produced food.

REFERENCES

Briefel, Ronette R., Mary Kay Crepinsek, Charlotte Cabili, Ander Wilson, and Philip Gleason. (2009). "School Food Environments and Practices Affect Dietary Behavior of US Public School Children," *Journal of American Dietetic Association 109*(suppl 1): S91-S 107.

Clark, Melissa, and Mary Kay Fox. (2009). "Nutritional Quality of the Diets of the US Public School Children and the Role of the School Meal Programs," *Journal of American Dietetic Association 109*(suppl 1): S44-S56.

Finkelstein, Daniel M., Elaine L. Hill, & Robert Whitaker. (2008). "School Food Environments and Policies in US Public Schools," *Pediatrics, 122*, e251-e259.

Fox, Mary Kay, Allison Hedley Dodd, Ander Wilson, and Philip Gleason. (2009). "Association Between School Food Environment and Practices and Body Mass Index of US Public School Children," *Journal of American Dietetic Association 109*(suppl 1): S108-S117.

Gordon, Anne, Elizabeth Condon, Melissa Clark, Karin Zeller, Elaine Hill, Ander Wilson, and Ronette Briefel. (2009). *School Nutrition Dietary Assessment Study-III: Public-Use File Documentation,* Version 2. February (.pdf file, unpublished).

Miller, Clare H. (2009). "Commentary: A Practice Perspective on the Third School Nutrition Dietary Assessment Study," *Journal of American Dietetic Association 109*(suppl 1): S14-S17.

U.S. Government Accountability Office. (2005). *School Meals Programs: Competitive Foods Are Widely Available and Generate Substantial Revenue for Schools.* GAO-05–563.

End Notes

[1] Whereas the majority of NSLP guidelines describe minimum values for essential nutrients, the guidelines for fat and saturated fat suggest maximum values, as a share of calories.

[2] For space considerations, we made a choice between using meals that are offered by schools (referred to in SNDA-III as "offered") versus those that are then chosen by students (or "served"). We chose "served" for the reasons mentioned. But we also conducted the analysis using the "offered" version of the variable, and the results were very similar. That work is available upon request from cnewman@ers. usda.gov.

[3] Foods and beverages were classified as low-nutrient, energy-dense (LNED) items if they were low in nutrients but high in energy or caloric density per unit volume or mass, or were defined as foods of minimal nutritional value by USDA school meal regulations. Sugar-

sweetened beverages and the following solid food categories were considered to be LNED items: (1) higher fat baked goods, including muffins and desserts such as cakes, cookies, and brownies; (2) dairy-based desserts (e.g., ice cream); (3) candy (all types) and sweetened gum; (4) french fries and similar potato products; and (5) high-fat chips and other salty snacks (e.g., potato chips, corn chips) (Gordon et al., 2009).

[4] Wellness policies are policies that are formed by local stakeholders (e.g., parents, students, interested health and school professionals) in an effort to im-prove school nutrition. In 2004, Congress required school food authorities to implement "local wellness policies" to improve nutrition policies with local input.

[5] "Farm to school" is a generic term that refers to any local or State-level program that links local or regional farmers directly to school food services.

[6] The U.S. Department of Defense's (DOD) Fresh Fruit and Vegetable Program is a program through which USDA commodity funds are usedfor reimbursable school meal food purchases in the DOD's procurement network, which has superior access to fresh fruits and vegetables.

In: Meals in School: Issues and Impacts   ISBN: 978-1-61209-127-3
Editors: Dayna A. Michalka et al.   © 2011 Nova Science Publishers, Inc.

Chapter 4

BEHAVIORAL ECONOMIC CONCEPTS TO ENCOURAGE HEALTHY EATING IN SCHOOL CAFETERIAS: EXPERIMENTS AND LESSONS FROM COLLEGE STUDENTS

David R. Just, Brian Wansink,
Lisa Mancino and Joanne Guthrie

ABSTRACT

Changing small factors that influence consumer choice may lead to healthier eating within controlled settings, such as school cafeterias. This chapter describes a behavioral experiment in a college cafeteria to assess the effects of various payment options and menu selection methods on food choices. The results indicate that payment options, such as cash or debit cards, can significantly affect food choices. College students using a card that prepaid only for healthful foods made more nutritious choices than students using either cash or general debit cards. How and when individuals select their food can also influence food choices. College students who preselected their meals from a menu board made significantly different food choices than students who ordered their meals while viewing the foods in line.

Keywords: Behavioral economics, healthy eating, diet quality, food choices, school meal programs, experimental economics, ERS, USDA.

ACKNOWLEDGMENTS

The authors greatly appreciate the thoughtful review suggestions from Jay Bhattacharya, Stanford University School of Medicine; Karen Cullen, Baylor College of Medicine; and Katherine Ralston, Economic Research Service (ERS). We also thank Linda Hatcher for editorial expertise and layout and Susan DeGeorge for the cover design.

SUMMARY

Poor diet quality, overconsumption, and inactivity can lead to poor health. Even with the plethora of weight-loss programs and diet books currently available, diet-related health conditions like obesity and diabetes continue to rise. Traditional economic analyses seem inadequate to explain why so many people choose risky health behaviors. Consequently, some researchers are turning to behavioral economics, which tries to explain why people act as they do and what incentives can modify behavior.

What Is the Issue?

Experiments have shown that the eating environment, such as the social atmosphere, the presence and level of distractions, or even lighting, can affect people's food choices and how much they eat. Some of those same cues can also be used to help individuals make healthier food choices. Finding successful ways to promote healthier food choices could be an important tool for the school meals programs, for example, which aim to strike a balance between meeting the dietary needs of students who are undernourished and encouraging healthy diets and body weight. Cafeteria administrators are in a unique position to control many of the elements that have been shown to influence food choice. By understanding how these behavioral interventions influence food choice and diet quality, managers of school and workplace cafeterias can devise possible strategies to promote healthy eating. This chapter describes a behavioral experiment in a college cafeteria, which assessed the effects of various menu selection methods and payment options on food choices. The experiment was designed to apply within the context of any cafeteria—whether college, work, or secondary school.

What Did the Study Find?

College students who preselected their meals from a menu board before seeing them did not always make healthier food choices than students who made their selections in line where they could see the food. In fact, viewing led to significantly greater consumption of healthier foods—salad and turkey sandwiches—and significantly less consumption of less healthy foods—French fries and caffeine. Viewing brownies, however, also significantly increased brownie consumption. The impact of viewing different foods may have more to do with how attractive they are than how healthy they are.

Students who participated in the experiment could pay for their meals in one of three ways—cash, prepaid cards to be used for any menu item (unrestricted debit cards), or prepaid cards to be used for more healthful items only (restricted debit cards). Their payment method affected the amount of money they spent on meals. Those using cash spent more on average than those who used an unrestricted debit card. Students using the restricted debit card spent the least on less nutritious items, whereas those using the unrestricted card spent the most on these foods.

The payment option significantly affected the types of foods chosen as well. College students paying with cash made healthier food choices than those paying with an unrestricted debit card, who were significantly more likely to purchase a brownie and a soda but less likely to buy skim milk and healthful side items and desserts. Parting with cash appeared to force more cognizant decisionmaking. Students using restricted cards made significantly healthier choices than students paying with either cash or unrestricted cards. In many cases, these differences were prominent and suggest that it is possible to change behavior by altering payment methods used for different foods.

Students using the unrestricted debit card consumed significantly more calories than students using either cash or the restricted card, with those using the restricted card consuming the fewest calories. Not only did the number of calories differ by payment method, the calories derived from healthful foods varied as well. Although those using the unrestricted card consumed the most calories, they consumed the least amount of calories from more nutritious foods. Those using the restricted card consumed the fewest calories overall but consumed more calories from more nutritious foods. Students using the restricted card also consumed significantly less added sugar, total fat, saturated fat, and caffeine than those who used the unrestricted card.

How Was the Study Conducted?

This chapter presents results from an experiment comparing the effects of various behavioral intervention strategies on the food choices of college students. Participants in the experiment were recruited from Cornell University. The experiment's participants used three types of payment options and two different meal selection methods.

INTRODUCTION: WHAT ARE THE MERITS OF USING BEHAVIORAL CUES TO INFLUENCE FOOD CHOICE?

Consistent overconsumption, poor diet quality, and inactivity are widely recognized as factors that can lead to severely poor health conditions. And the continued popularity of weight-loss programs and diet books indicate that individuals are interested in improving their own health and wellness. Public information programs like the *Dietary Guidelines for Americans* and mandatory nutrition labels have also been in existence for years. Yet the incidences of diet-related health conditions like obesity and diabetes continue to rise. So, why do poor diet and lifestyle choices persist among nearly all segments of the population?

Traditional economic analysis that emphasizes the role of prices, income, and time-consistent preferences seem to inadequately explain why so many people choose to take on these risky health behaviors. Consequently, more researchers are turning to behavioral economics, which identifies predictable and systematic contradictions to many standard assumptions of economics. For example, the idea of complete rationality is challenged by repeated observance of cognitive biases that can lead to systematic errors in decisionmaking.

A growing body of research also suggests that today's food environment is replete with instances in which these biases can influence dietary choice. Other behavioral studies show that environmental factors seem to strongly affect the amount of food people eat. In particular, both the eating and food environments affect consumption volume by setting consumption norms (an indication of how much people should consume) and inhibiting monitoring accuracy. Thus, these subtle cues can have large impacts on consumption volume, often without the individual being aware of their effect (see Wansink, 2006, for a complete review of the literature on consumption volume and the eating environment).

Behavioral studies on dietary choice also suggest that subtle changes in the food environment may help to leverage some of these cognitive biases and offer novel ways for improving diets and health (Just, Mancino, and Wansink, 2007). A key advantage of behavioral interventions is that, in theory, they can be targeted to improve food choices among individuals who behave contrary to their own long-term health objectives without reducing the welfare of individuals who feel they do make optimal choices. As such, these changes have the added benefit of being less paternalistic (Camerer et al., 2003; Sunstein and Thaler, 2003). Another advantage of leveraging behavioral influences is that they may require only slight modifications to existing programs.

To gauge the efficacy of behavioral economic tools in shaping food choices and eating environments, this chapter summarizes the results of a behavioral experiment designed to apply within the context of a cafeteria—college, work, or secondary school. For these experiments, we focus on when diners select their meals and how they pay for them because these elements are common to most cafeterias. Understanding how slight modifications to payment and selection methods may influence food choice and diet quality can be used to augment specific policies, such as work and school well¬ness programs that are meant to combat obesity and promote healthy eating among students or employees.

For example, knowing how changes in payment options affect food choices can identify specific ways to help individuals make choices that are better aligned with their own dietary goals and intentions. Further, by understanding how expenditures may vary with payment and selection options, behavioral interventions can be designed to encourage better eating without necessarily reducing profitability. Note, however, that this is a small-scale study, the results of which should not be interpreted as widely generalizable. Pilot studies within cafeterias would be needed to accurately assess the full costs, benefits, and feasibility of the interventions discussed in this study.

In the following section, we provide some background information on the theory and literature used to develop our research hypotheses. (For a more detailed treatment of the literature on behavioral economics as it relates to nutrition assistance programs, see Just, Mancino, and Wansink, 2007.) We then describe the experiment design, sample population, and findings. We conclude with implications for possible policy interventions and directions for future research.

BEHAVIORAL STUDIES SHOW THAT *WHEN* *YOU CHOOSE* CAN AFFECT YOUR SELECTION

One of the most widely documented anomalies in behavioral studies is that individuals tend to view the tradeoff between immediate consumption and future consumption as having a larger impact on satisfaction than if this same tradeoff were between two future adjacent periods (Laibson, 2004). This tendency implies that individuals are more sensitive to time delays that occur sooner rather than later. As such, one's willingness to make sacrifices in terms of limiting salt, calories, and fat for better health in the future would be lower if one were considering limiting salt, calories, and fat right now versus limiting salt, calories, and fat tomorrow.

This behavior, sometimes referred to *present-biased preferences,* can cause a rift between long-term objectives and short-term desires and, in turn, may lead to seemingly inconsistent choices. Other behavioral studies have found that specific situations and behavioral cues may further bias preferences towards the present. For example, certain visceral influences, like feeling hungry or stressed, are also associated with more seemingly impulsive behavior (Loewenstein, 2004; Polivy et al., 1986). Simply seeing a food can also lead to unplanned consumption (Boon et al., 1998; Cornell, Rodin, and Weingarten, 1989). Distracting environments can also exacerbate present-biased preferences and cause individuals to make less healthful choices (Shiv and Fedorikhin, 1999).

Behavioral studies, however, show that individuals who commit to their decision before being confronted with distractions, visceral influences, or the promise of immediate gratification are less likely to exhibit present-biased preferences. These studies also show that individuals can improve their longrun well-being through some commitment technology, such as 401k plans, that set limits on current consumption levels. For example, Thaler and Benartzi (2004) found that savings rates increased dramatically when employees were offered a plan where a specified fraction of their future pay increases were automatically diverted into a savings account. Applying this finding to school or work cafeterias suggests that allowing individuals to precommit to healthful meal options before they consume the food likely will improve the healthfulness of their meal choices.

How You Pay Can Also Influence
What you Choose

In most cafeterias, individuals have the option of using cash or some form of credit, debit, or prepaid card. At colleges, students typically enroll in a specific, prepaid meal plan, where a meal card functions as a prepaid debit card or entitles students to a preset number of visits. It is becoming increasingly more common for parents to prepay for meals in high, middle, and grade schools as well, where students receive meal cards that are used to debit the account when they go through the cafeteria line each day. These prepaid cards are also used by students receiving free and reduced-price meals, minimizing any appearance of differences in payment between them and students who are paying full price (Bland, 2004). In most systems, the cash that parents deposit into these prepaid accounts can be used for a la carte items as well as meals provided by the U.S. Department of Agriculture (USDA), although some systems offer parents the opportunity to prohibit a la carte purchases. Students still have the option of paying cash.

This choice of using a prepaid card or cash presents individuals with two different payment options. While both are denominated in dollars, cash not spent on cafeteria meals can be spent on other items either immediately or sometime in the future. Alternatively, money on the prepaid account can be used only on food, until some date in the future when excess money is returned. Because the use of prepaid dollars is limited (both by time and choice), these dollars have less value to the consumer than cash in their pockets that can be used for anything at any time. Thus, putting $20 on a prepaid account may lead to greater food consumption than $20 in cash. This *discount effect* suggests that, compared with cash, prepayment cards may lead to greater spending on food and, thus, greater consumption volume.

Prepayment is also a form of commitment device. Findings from the behavioral and experimental economics literature indicate that allowing individuals to prepay for certain items may also tighten the link between intentions and behaviors. Contrary to standard economic models, individuals exhibit a "flat-rate bias," where they undervalue fixed costs, relative to variable costs (Thaler, 2004). For example, health club members typically choose to pay for their gym membership on a monthly or annual basis, even when a per use fee would have lower total costs (DellaVigna and Malmendier, 2002).

An implication of a flat-rate bias is that, when only certain items can be selected using prepayment, those items will be chosen with greater frequency compared with items that can be purchased only with cash. Thus, if only the more healthful menu items can be selected using prepayment, then individuals using this prepayment method would be more likely to make significantly healthier food choices.

Behavioral studies show that individuals also tend to categorize their income into mental accounts, earmarking it for specific purposes or specifying that it be used within a certain timeframe (Thaler, 1980; Shefrin and Thaler, 2004). Mental accounting suggests that a prepaid card for only healthful menu items may also provide cues about how much money should be spent on healthful items. As such, the combined effect of flat-rate biases and mental accounting should increase the healthfulness of meals chosen by students who have prepaid for healthful menu items.

Another implication of a flat-rate bias is that, because of these different levels of valuation, if one has prepaid into a flexible lunch account, he or she is likely to be less sensitive to variations in price compared with students who pay with cash. Thus, prepayment can reduce awareness of the cost of foods, creating less discriminating consumers. If all foods in a school cafeteria are available for purchase on this account, people should behave differently, being more willing to spend extra money on unnecessary foods or to buy more food, in terms of portion sizes or variety, because prepaid funds are less fungible.

Finally, prepayment for all items may increase sensitivity to environmental factors by reducing the general level of cognition and encouraging impulse buying. Thus, students using an unrestricted prepaid card likely will spend more money on "frivolous" items compared with students using cash or restricted debit cards.

TESTING OUR HYPOTHESES: EXPERIMENT DESIGN, SAMPLE, AND SETTING

Observations from behavioral economic literature on the relationship among food choices, the timing of these choices, and payment options suggest a number of hypotheses related to school meal environments. As such, the food choice experiments in this study were designed to test the following hypotheses:

- Individuals who preselect their meals from a menu board are likely to make healthier food choices than those who make their selection in line.
- Individuals using prepayment cards are likely to spend more on cafeteria meals than those who pay with cash.
- Individuals using a restricted prepaid card will make healthier food choices than those using either cash or an unrestricted prepaid card.
- Individuals using an unrestricted prepaid card will spend less money on nutritious items than individuals using cash or restricted debit cards.

To test our hypotheses, the experiment included three types of payment options and two different selection methods (table 1). For selecting foods, individuals either chose their foods at the point of purchase or precommitted to a choice made beforehand from a menu. The menus used in these experiments listed the name of food and beverage choices within each category and their corresponding price (table 2). The three payment options were prepaid cards that could be used for any menu item (prepaid, unrestricted), prepaid cards that could be used for healthful items only (prepaid, restricted), and cash.

The menu items chosen for this experiment were typical of cafeteria menus and familiar to participants. Under each heading, we included an equal number of more nutritious (those with a green dot) and less nutritious options. Prices were taken from existing menus at Cornell University dining facilities and rounded to the nearest half dollar.

Table 1. Experimental treatments

Treatments	Prepaid		Cash only
	Unrestricted: All menu items are eligible	Restricted: Only healthful items are eligible	
Preselection: Foods are chosen off menu before consumption	Sample size: 52	Sample size: 55	Sample size: 49
Selection onsite: Foods chosen in line	Sample size: 58	Sample size: 62	Sample size: 47

Source: Economic Research Service, USDA.

Participants for the experiments were recruited from Cornell University, primarily from an introductory business course (74.9 percent) and consisted mostly of freshmen business students. Of those reporting their age, 51 percent were ages 19 or younger. Additional participants walked on or were brought by other participants. A potential drawback of using a convenience sample of college students is that the results may not be widely generalizable to other population groups of interest. This drawback is especially problematic if the convenience sample does not regularly consume the goods or services in question. In this case, however, the goods in question were foods offered in a school cafeteria and that college students consume regularly. While college and high school students may behave differently in terms of social norms, it is not clear a priori how this would systematically affect food choices. In addition, cafeteria habits could be well ingrained by the time they reach college. That is, because students are used to the cafeteria context (in elementary, middle, and high school), they already have ingrained behavior that would not change much in the college context. Also, efforts were made to increase the realism of the study. The experimental sessions took place in a section of one of the dining facilities at Cornell University where the layout of the room and presentation of the food was closely controlled so that differences in behavior would not be ascribed to inadvertent changes in presentation. This section, which we refer to as the cafeteria, was separated from the rest of the eating facility by temporary walls made of opaque material.

All experimental procedures were reviewed and approved by Cornell University's Institutional Review Board. Each participant was assigned to a prepayment treatment and asked to participate in two lunch sessions 1 week apart, the first sessions requiring the participant to preorder from a menu board without seeing the food and the second requiring them to order while viewing the food. A total of 191 students participated in the study—167 participated in the first session, 156 participated in the second, which gave a total of 323 observed orders, where 109 were from students who participated in both sessions. The variation in participation allows us to discern how the design of the experiment may have influenced behavior. In particular, because those participating in both sessions always participated in the preorder condition first, this experience may have had some influence on behavior in the second session. For example, having already tried some of the foods may have led one to choose based on taste recall rather than the aesthetics of the food.

Table 2. Menu choices

Choices	Item	Price
Entrees	Bacon cheeseburger • Chicken breast sandwich • Turkey sandwich Chicken fingers	$5.00 $5.00 $4.50 $4.00
Sides	French fries • Baked potato chips • Salad Macaroni and cheese	$1.00 $1.00 $2.00 $2.50
Desserts	• Peaches Brownie	$1.00 $1.50
Drinks	• Skim milk Soda • Bottled water	$1.00 $1.00 $1.50

• = More nutritious.
Source: Economic Research Service, USDA.

A standard script was read to each group before entering the cafeteria. Each participant was given a combination of $20 in either prepayment money or in cash each time they participated. In both prepayment conditions, participants were given $10 on the prepaid card and $10 in cash to ensure that participants were not truly restricted in their lunch purchases. For example, a participant in the healthy card condition could have spent cash to purchase any combination of entrée, side, dessert, and drink. Rather, the healthy card only suggests a restriction by drawing attention to the tradeoffs between current and future consumption. In the cash condition, participants were given $20 in cash. To track individual purchases, all participants were given an identification card that was the size of a standard credit card.

Participants in the prepaid conditions were informed that the card would serve as a debit card upon which they had been given $10. They were informed that all cash not used that day could be kept and all money left on the card after the second week could be picked up at a separate location on campus after a specified date 2 weeks after the close of the experiment. All participants were informed that more money would be given for the second session and that balances on the debit cards would carry over. Finally, participants assigned to the prepayment—healthy session were given plastic cards (identical to standard credit cards) with circular green stickers placed on the nonmagnetic face. The menu they viewed had a similar green sticker placed next to each of the healthy items (table 2) as well as on the name plates placed in front of items in the cafeteria line. They were informed that the debit card could be used only for these items and that they could still use cash for other menu items.

Participants in the preselection condition were instructed to choose their food selections from the menu board and fill out an order card before entering the cafeteria. This order was then given to a researcher who would accompany the participant into the food line and give the order card to those preparing the food orders. Alternatively, when ordering from sight, participants would fill out the same card in line while viewing all the menu options. In this case, the cards were handed directly from the participant to those preparing the dishes. We tracked the orders of all participants and collected sociodemographic information by survey after lunch was completed.

EXPERIMENTAL RESULTS

In this section, we report the differences in food choices, calories consumed, nutrient intake, and total expenditures by selection method and payment mechanism. To measure actual consumption, each participant's order was recorded. His or her plate was then weighed at the end of the meal. The difference between the average weight for each item and the end weight of each individual's plate was then taken to be the amount consumed in grams. For each outcome—food choice, calories consumed, nutrient intake, and total expenditures—we first report the mean intake by treatment and whether the mean differed significantly from the other treatment(s). Summary statistics for the entire sample are reported in table 3. Here, more nutritious foods are defined as those that were included on the green-dotted menu (chicken breast sandwich, turkey sandwich, baked potato chips, salad, peaches, skim milk, and bottled water) and the less nutritious foods are those without a green dot (bacon cheeseburger, chicken fingers, French fries, macaroni and cheese, brownie, and soda).

Table 3. Summary Statistics—All Treatments

Variable	Definition and units	Mean	Standard deviation
Males	Percent of sample	0.4829	0.5005
Weight	Pounds	154.6	31.84
Body Mass Index	Height/weight^2	23.38	3.434
Hours since last eaten	Hours	6.959	5.807
Bacon cheeseburger	Percent of sample that chose menu item	0.1615	0.3686
Chicken breast sandwich	Percent of sample that chose menu item	0.2671	0.4431
Turkey sandwich	Percent of sample that chose menu item	0.2391	0.4344
Chicken fingers	Percent of sample that chose menu item	0.1863	0.3900
Salad	Percent of sample that chose menu item	0.1957	0.3973
Baked potato chips	Percent of sample that chose menu item	0.2019	0.4020
Macaroni and cheese	Percent of sample that chose menu item	0.1308	0.3378
French fries	Percent of sample that chose menu item	0.2112	0.4088
Brownie	Percent of sample that chose menu item	0.0590	0.2360
Peaches	Percent of sample that chose menu item	0.2298	0.4214
Skim milk	Percent of sample that chose menu item	0.1242	0.3396
Soft drink	Percent of sample that chose menu item	0.2516	0.4346
Bottled water	Percent of sample that chose menu item	0.4068	0.4920
Calories	Calories consumed at that meal	633.3	296.0
Calories from more nutritious foods	Calories from "healthy" (green-dotted) foods	276.4	232.3
Calories from less nutritious foods	Calories from "unhealthy" foods	358.2	373.8
Added sugar	Grams	7.138	6.937
Total fat	Grams	27.23	17.03
Saturated fat	Grams	7.572	6.173
Percent calories from fat	Percent	37.04	20.86
Percent calories from caturated fat	Percent	10.48	09.14
Sodium	Milligrams	1,212	669.4
Caffeine	Milligrams	10.37	17.64
Expenditures	Dollars spent at that meal	6.508	2.214
Sample size		322	

Source: Economic Research Service, USDA.

Table 4. Mean height, weight, gender, and hours since last eaten by treatment

Factors	In line	Menu board	Cash	Unrestricted card	Restricted card
Males:					
Mean	0.47	0.471	0.50	0.50	0.4615
Standard deviation	(0.501)	(0.501)	(0.503)	(0.502)	(0.501)
Weight (pounds):					
Mean	155.69	153.44	150.76	161.33	151.45
Standard deviation	(32.10)	(31.51)	(29.25)	(32.66)	(32.36)
Body Mass Index:					
Mean	23.41	23.34	22.78	24.29	23.00
Standard deviation	(3.422)	(3.448)	(3.349)	(3.445)	(3.342)
Hours since last meal:					
Mean	7.08	6.80	7.24	7.64	6.103
Standard deviation	(6.038)	(5.557)	(5.745)	(6.192)	(5.421)
Sample size	167	152	95	109	117

Source: Economic Research Service, USDA.

The Effect of Preselection on Food Choice, Diet Quality, and Expenditures

Preselecting foods before seeing them did not always lead to healthier food choices. Past studies found that precommitment mechanisms helped individuals assuage the effect of present-biased preferences to make decisions that were more harmonious with future well-being. However, in this experiment, we found that the effect of ordering in line while viewing the food was nuanced and not so simple as "viewing drives one to order less healthy foods." In fact, viewing led to significantly greater consumption of salad and turkey sandwiches and significantly less consumption of French fries, chicken sandwiches, and caffeine. Viewing brownies increased their consumption significantly. Thus, viewing different foods can have a varied impact that may have more to do with how attractive they are than how healthy they are. Table 5 presents differences in average consumption for foods preselected while viewing a menu board and selected in line while viewing the food.

The Effect of Payment Mechanism on Food Choice, Diet Quality, and Expenditures

We find that the frequency with which certain foods are ordered significantly differs by payment type (table 6, Figures 1a-c). In particular, individuals using an unrestricted debit card are significantly more likely to purchase a brownie (about 25 percent more likely) and a soda (about 27 percent more likely) but less likely to buy skim milk (about 7 percent less likely) than those using cash. Individuals using the unrestricted card were also more likely to buy less healthful (though similarly priced) side items and desserts than those using cash. In general, a prepaid card may change an individual's valuation of the dollar with respect to particular foods. However, note that very little difference is observed for entrees and both groups purchased water at about the same rate.

Behavior when using the restricted debit card was markedly different compared with behavior when using either cash or the unrestricted cards. In every case, except for the turkey sandwich and skim milk, green-dotted items were consumed significantly more under the restricted treatment. In many cases, these differences are prominent and suggest that it is possible to change behavior by altering payment methods used for different foods.

Comparing the restricted and unrestricted debit card treatments, the differences again are stark, with healthy items being consumed about twice as often in most cases. The restricted card cuts consumption significantly for most unhealthy items, the exceptions being the brownie and macaroni and cheese. However, these unhealthy items were seldom consumed under either treatment.

The differences among food choices, by payment treatment, also led to significant differences in diet quality. In terms of calories, those using the unrestricted debit card consumed significantly more calories than either the cash or restricted treatment groups, with those using the restricted card consuming the fewest calories at that meal. Not only did the total number of calories differ by payment method, the calories derived from healthful foods varied as well (Figure 2). Although those using the unrestricted card consumed the most calories at lunch, they got the fewest calories from more nutritious foods. In comparison, those using the restricted card consumed the fewest calories overall but consumed more calories from more nutritious foods. Compared with the individuals who used the unrestricted card, those using the restricted card also consumed significantly less added sugar, total fat, saturated fat, and caffeine.

Table 5. Mean differences in consumption and expenditures by selection treatment

Food choice	In line		Menu board		Within subject differences (in line–menu board)	
	Mean	Standard deviation	Mean	deviation Standard	Mean	Standard deviation
Bacon cheeseburger	0.1667	0.3739	0.1557	0.3637	0.0227	0.4534
Chicken breast sandwich**	0.3269	0.4706	0.2096	0.4082	0.1061	0.51 33
Turkey sandwich**	0.1923	0.4114	0.2874	0.4539	-0.0758	0.51 87
Chicken fingers	0.1987	0.4003	0.1737	0.3799	-0.01 52	0.5240
Salad**	0.1474	0.3557	0.2395	0.4281	-0.0909	0.4532
Baked potato chips	0.2308	0.4227	0.1796	0.3850	0.0303	0.4613
Macaroni and cheese	0.1538	0.3620	0.1084	0.3119	0.0229	0.3816
French fries*	0.2500	0.4344	0.1737	0.3799	0.0455	0.4764
Brownie***·†	0.01 92	0.1378	0.0958	0.2952	-0.0758	0.2930
Peaches	0.2179	0.4142	0.2395	0.4281	-0.0076	0.4004
Skim milk	0.1218	0.3281	0.1257	0.3502	0.000	0.3027
Soft drink	0.2243	0.41 85	0.2754	0.4481	-0.0530	0.3771
Bottled water	0.4038	0.4922	0.41 32	0.4939	0.0076	0.4539
Calories	643.99	295.44	623.23	297.04	-2.8230	258.72
Calories from more nutritious foods	282.99	239.22	270.84	225.75	14.4091	235.78
Calories from less nutritious foods	362.56	378.20	351.90	370.66	-13.8779	345.91
Percent Calories from fat	38.61	22.75	34.80	20.28	01.98	24.14
Percent calories from saturated fat	10.93	10.23	13.17	23.67	-2.87	24.90
Added sugar (grams)	6.50	6.10	7.74	7.61	-0.4918	5.6485
Total fat (grams)	26.35	17.59	26.17	16.48	1.7804	16.6218
Saturated fat (grams)	7.87	6.34	7.30	5.97	0.4212	6.7961
Sodium (milligrams)	1,246.65	704.14	1,179.98	635.25	45.7224	731.75
Caffeine (milligrams)**	9.11	16.95	11.56	18.24	-2.4688	14.8186
Expenditures (dollars)	6.14	2.40	6.41	2.03	0.00	1.6939
Sample size	156		167		132	

*,**,***Mean of menu board and in-line selection differ by 10, 5, and 1 percent using within-subject variation.

†,‡ Differences are significant at the 10- and 5-percent level after using the Bonferroni corrected p-values.

Source: Economic Research Service, USDA.

Table 6. Differences in mean consumption and expenditures by payment method

Food choice	Cash		Unrestricted card		Restricted card	
	Mean	Standard deviation	Mean	Standard deviation	Mean	Standard deviation
Bacon cheeseburger++,^^,‡	0.1771	0.3837	0.2364	0.4268	0.0769	0.2676
Chicken breast sandwich++,^^,†	0.2396	0.4291	0.1818	0.3875	0.3675	0.4842
Turkey sandwich^	0.2500	0.4353	0.1818	0.4105	0.2906	0.4560
Chicken fingers+++,‡,^^,‡	0.2604	0.4412	0.2636	0.4426	0.0513	0.2215
Salad+++,‡,^^	0.1146	0.3202	0.1455	0.3542	0.3077	0.4635
Baked potato chips+++,‡,†	0.0938	0.2930	0.1636	0.3716	0.3333	0.4734
Macaroni and cheese+	0.1875	0.3924	0.1091	0.3132	0.1034	0.3059
French fries+,^^	0.2292	0.4225	0.2727	0.4474	0.1368	0.3451
Brownie*	0.0313	0.1749	0.0909	0.2888	0.0513	0.2215
Peaches++,^^,‡	0.1875	0.3924	0.1455	0.3542	0.3419	0.4764
Skim milk**,^^	0.1563	0.3650	0.0545	0.2281	0.1624	0.3930
Soft drink***,‡,^^,‡	0.2188	0.4156	0.4182	0.4955	0.1197	0.3260
Bottled water+++,‡,^^	0.3229	0.4700	0.3636	0.4832	0.5214	0.5017
Calories++,^^,‡	644.37	275.00	692.14	306.64	568.90	292.27
Calories from more nutritious foods**,+++,‡,^^,‡	248.88	198.27	192.36	222.97	377.14	230.83
Calories from less nutritious foods**,+++,‡,^^,‡	397.43	346.19	502.01	377.42	190.55	326.90
Added sugar (grams)***,‡,^^	6.0659	6.3776	9.0728	7.9937	6.2067	5.9092
Total fat (grams)+++,‡,^^,‡	30.4493	17.1860	30.0914	17.4616	21.8740	15.2179

Table 6. (Continued)

Food choice	Cash		Unrestricted card		Restricted card	
	Mean	**Standard deviation**	**Mean**	**Standard deviation**	**Mean**	**Standard deviation**
Saturated fat (grams)[+++,‡,∧∧∧,÷]	8.8062	6.3338	8.2227	6.5460	5.9387	5.3173
Percent calories from fat[+++,‡,∧]	41.64	20.16	37.44	21.00	32.84	20.63
Percent calories from saturated fat[++]	12. 23	09.15	10.42	92.13	09.08	08.88
Sodium (milligrams)*,[+]	1,320.766	643.611	1,165.417	723.959	1,166.808	631 .227
Caffeine (milligrams)****,[+,‡,∧∧∧,÷,‡]	8.91 44	16.7695	17.3058	20.1072	5.0487	13.3341
Expenditures (dollars)[+,∧∧]	$6.53	2.26	$6.33	1.96	$6.66	2.40
Sample size	96		110		117	

*, **, ***Mean of cash treatment and unrestricted card treatment differ by 1 0, 5, and 1 percent.

+, ++, +++Mean of cash treatment and restricted card treatment differ by 10, 5, and 1 percent.

∧, ∧∧, ∧∧∧ Mean of restricted and unrestricted card treatment differ by 10, 5, and 1 percent.

†,‡ Differences are significant at the 10- and 5-percent level after using the Bonferroni corrected p-values.

Source: Economic Research Service, USDA.

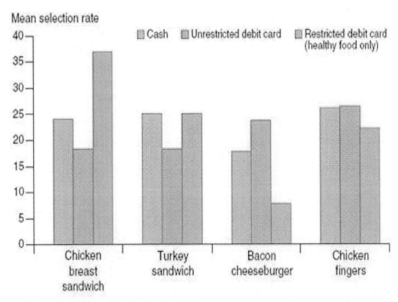

Source: Economic Research Service, USDA.

Figure 1a. Variations in food choice by payment type—entrees Mean selection rate

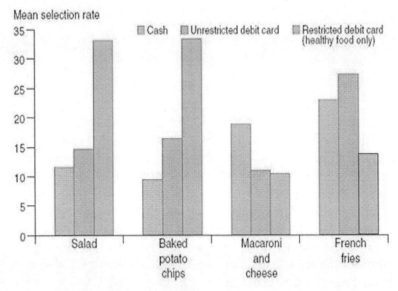

Source: Economic Research Service, USDA.

Figure 1b. Variations in food choice by payment type—sides Mean selection rate

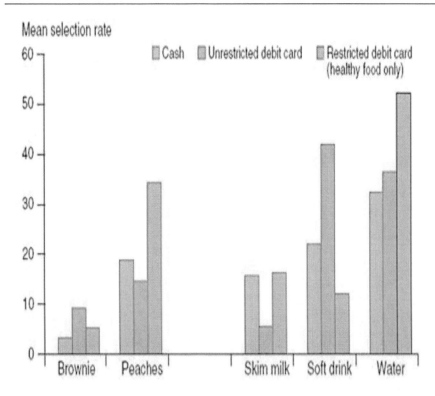

Source: Economic Research Service, USDA.

Figure 1c. Variations in food choice by payment type—desserts and sides Mean selection rate

Our results show no greater spending when using unrestricted prepaid cards compared with using cash. In fact, individuals using cash spent more on average than those who used an unrestricted prepaid card (Figure 3). However, individuals using the restricted card spent the least on unhealthy items, whereas those using the unrestricted card spent the most on these foods. The maximum amount spent was $16.50, with an average of $6.51. In fact, only one participant from the combined cash and restricted card experiment spent more than the $10 given in cash. Thus, only this participant could have been constrained in his or her choice by the funds given. The average amount spent in either card treatment was $6.51, and less than 1 percent of individuals spent all of their money on the card in a single lunch.

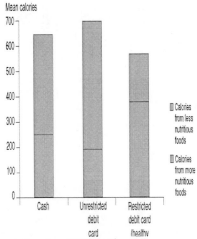

Source: Economic Research Service, USDA. Figure 3

Figure 2. Differences in caloric intake by payment type Mean calories

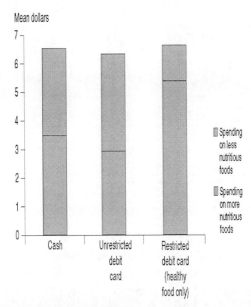

Source: Economic Research Service, USDA.

Figure 3. Differences in spending by payment type Mean dollars

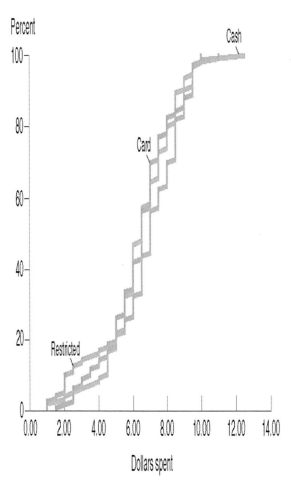

Source: Economic Research Service, USDA.

Figure 4. Cumulative distribution of spending for cash and debit card treatments

Figure 4 displays the cumulative distribution of spending by the three different payment methods. Comparing those using cash to those using the unrestricted debit card, the distributions are nearly identical, except that no one using the card spent above $10. One explanation for this result could be that the amount on the card suggested a limit on spending that would not otherwise exist, curbing the consumption of those on the upper tail. In fact, no individual spent any cash when given an unrestricted debit card

However, little weight should be placed on differences in the tails of distributions, and further tests would be needed to determine whether this result is robust to altered levels of card endowments.

When faced with the restricted debit card, individuals spent an average of 13 cents more than they did when using cash. Unlike the unrestricted treatment, here we observe that the spending distribution for the restricted treatment diverges from the cash treatment, with more mass placed on the tails of the distribution. Again, we note that individuals using the card tended not to spend more than $10. In this case, the effect is clearly due to the spending norm suggested by the amount on the debit card. Most participants spent some cash in addition to the money spent on a debit card (on average $1.04).

MEASURING TREATMENT EFFECTS: HOW MUCH OF THE VARIATION IN FOOD CHOICE IS DUE TO PAYMENT EFFECT?

Testing for differences in mean values among payment and preselection options suggests that these treatments do correlate with different food choices. However, it is important to recognize that other factors, such as an individual's gender, Body Mass Index (BMI), or how long he or she had gone between meals, may also affect his or her food choices.

Thus, for a more precise measure of the effect of each treatment, we use propensity matching scores to estimate how much expenditures and nutrient intake respond to each treatment, while holding these factors constant. In particular, we use the matching estimation procedure developed by Abadie, Drukker, Herr, Imbens (2004), which matches outcomes between treated observations to those in the control based on a vector of independent variables. Matches are determined by minimizing Euclidean distance, and a sample of nearest matches are drawn for estimation of the treatment effect. See Abadie, Drukker, Herr, and Imbens (2001) for details.

After controlling for these factors, we still find that our results hold (table 7). Namely, individuals using the unrestricted card consumed 95 more calories, 2 more grams of added sugars, 7 more grams of fat, 2 more grams of saturated fat, and 11 more milligrams of caffeine than individuals using the restricted debit card. Over time, these seemingly small differences could lead to substantial changes in diet quality, body weight, and health.

Table 7. Mean Effect Controlling for Body Mass Index, Gender, and Hours since Last Meal

Item	Cash versus unrestricted		Cash versus restricted		Unrestricted versus restricted	
	Mean	Standard deviation	Mean	Standard deviation	Mean	Standard deviation
Calories	21.3002	52.3336	76.45016*	45.34302	94.4898**	48.8895
Calories from more nutritious foods	102.0725***‡	34.5758	86.6949**	35.8072	198.0445***‡	34.7789
Calories from less nutritious foods	123.1275**	56.91 96	170.5736***‡	52.21 25	294.8636***‡	54.7064
Added sugar	2.961 1**	1.3731	0.3440	0.9638	2.2396*	1.2265
Total fat	2.3344	2.9570	8.4740***‡	2.6522	6.8768***†	2.5082
Saturated fat	1.1275	1.1311	2.9113***‡	0.9678	2.0220**	0.9455
Percent calories from fat	7.01*	4.02	9.82***†	3.56	6.38**	3.15
Percent calories from saturated fat	3.02*	1.86	3.77**	1.59	2.28*	1.41
Sodium	259.931**	124.093	193.369*	104.652	37.9986	105.659
Caffeine	9.6243***‡	3.1801	4.3701 *	2.3337	11.7405***‡	3.0359
Expenditures	0.5038	0.4112	0.2252	0.3718	0.3853	0.3771

*, **, ***Treatments differ by 10, 5, and 1 percent.

†, ‡Differences are significant at the 10- and 5-percent level after using the Bonferroni corrected p-values.

POSSIBLE POLICY IMPLICATIONS

While this study is on a small scale and the results should not be interpreted as widely generalizable, the results may have implications for environmental strategies for obesity protection. In particular schools may find these concepts useful as they strive to design wellness policies that would promote healthful food choices by students.

Schools participating in the National School Lunch Program (NSLP) receive cash and some commodities from USDA. In return, these schools provide free or reduced-price lunches to needy school children whose families meet the income cutoffs. National food consumption survey data indicate that many children choose foods high in saturated fat, sodium, and added sugars at the expense of fruits, vegetables, low-fat milk, and whole grains (Lin et al., 2001). In response, today's NSLP seeks to promote both adequate intake of healthful foods and limits on high-calorie, low-nutrient foods. Meals sold as part of the NSLP must meet Federal dietary standards, which include limits on fat and saturated fat (Oliveira, 2006; for a detailed account of the history, trends, and objectives of the NSLP, see Ralston et al., 2007).

However, most American schools choose to sell at least some foods and beverages that are not a part of the USDA school meal program (O'Toole et al., 2007). These foods and beverages are often labeled "competitive foods" because they compete with NSLP meals and have been criticized as being frequently high in calories, saturated fat, sodium, or sugars (O'Toole et al., 2007). A 2005 study of U.S. public schools found that, although less than half of all public schools have vending machines, nearly 80 percent of schools offer a la carte foods (Finkelstein, Hill, and Whitaker, 2008). This study also found that school food environments are less healthy among children in higher grade levels and that most secondary schools offer less nutritious foods through a la carte and vending machines sales. Competition with less nutritious options may result in decreased consumption of the healthier choices provided through USDA meals. The School Nutrition Dietary Assessment Study-III (SNDA-III) found that, although USDA school meals provided to all grade levels regularly include fruit or juice, only 32 percent of high school student participants reported consuming fruit at lunch compared with 55 percent of elementary school participants (Gordon et al., 2007).

To address current concerns about high-calorie, low-nutrient foods being sold in American schools, the Child Nutrition and WIC (Special Supplemental Nutrition Program for Women, Infants, and Children) Reauthorization Act of 2004 (Public Law 108-265) required that every school district participating in the NSLP, as of school year 2006-07, have a local school wellness policy. It is intended to be a tool to address obesity and promote healthy eating and physical activity through changes in school environments. Each district's wellness policy must provide assurances that school meals meet Federal guidelines; provide nutrition guidelines for all foods available at school; and specify goals for nutrition education, physical activity, and other school-based wellness activities. However, districts have flexibility as to the specific policies and guidelines they develop.

Suggested strategies for improving the choices of foods and beverages made by children and adolescents at school have included nutrition education, restricting sales of some items, or manipulating prices of a la carte items to encourage healthful choices (Story et al., 2006). While such intervention policies have been shown to influence food choice, psychological and behavioral tools may be as equally effective as these more traditional interventions (Just, Mancino, and Wansink, 2007).

Our research findings suggest that allowing individuals, or in the case of younger school-aged children, their parents, to prepay for a restricted set of approved foods may result in increased consumption of healthful foods. Depending on the infrastructure of the cafeteria, offering a restricted card along with an unrestricted card may be possible. How closely the results of this experiment resemble those in an actual cafeteria setting will depend heavily on how well individuals understand the debit card system and its potential impacts on diet quality.

It may also be important to evaluate which foods should be displayed when ordering and which should be hidden until after ordering has taken place. This choice should be based on the visual appeal of the items and their nutritional content. Thus, it may be useful for cafeterias to monitor the specific reactions to the foods they consider placing prominently. This effect can be fine tuned by tracking how sales of each item change with changes in product placement.

A key advantage of leveraging behavioral influences is that they may only require slight modifications to existing programs. Also, administrators of school food services are in a unique position to control many of the elements that have been shown to influence food choice, such as the order and way in which foods are presented, when they can be selected, and the actual eating environment. Results of this experiment suggest that placing limitations on items that can be purchased with prepaid debit cards improves the healthfulness of food choices. An advantage of such a system is that it could allow parents significant control over their child's purchases, without necessarily decreasing overall choice within a school. However, the interventions discussed in this study may be better suited for middle and high school meal programs. And of course, pilot studies within school cafeterias would be needed to accurately assess the full costs, benefits, and feasibility of these interventions.

REFERENCES

Abadie, Alberto, David Drukker, Jane Leber Herr, and Guido W. Imbens. (2004). "Implementing Matching Estimators for Average Treatment Effects in Stata," *The Stata Journal, 4(3)*, 290-31 1, StataCorp LP.

Abadie, Alberto, David Drukker, Jane Leber Herr, Guido, W. Imbens. (2001). "Implementing Matching Estimators for Average Treatment Effects in Stata," *The Stata Journal, 1(1)*, 1-18, StataCorp LP.

Bland, Karina. (2004). "Kids Using Debit Cards to Pay For School Lunch," *The Arizona Republic*, August 30, 2004, accessed at *https://www.mylunchmoney.com/azcentral.htm.*

Boon, B., Stroebe, W., Schut, H. & Jansen, A. (1998). "Food for Thought: Cognitive Regulation of Food Intake," *British Journal of Health Psychology, 3(1)*, 27-40.

Camerer, Colin, Samuel Issacharoff, George Loewenstein, Ted O'Donoghue, and Matthew Rabin. (2003). "Regulation for Conservatives: Behavioral Economics and the Case of 'Asymmetric Paternalism,'" *University of Pennsylvania Law Review, 151(3)*, 1211-54.

Cornell, C. E., Rodin, J. & Weingarten, H. (1989). "Stimulus-Induced Eating When Satiated," *Physiology and Behavior, 45(4)*, 695-704.

DellaVigna, S. & Malmendier, U. (2002). *"Overestimating Self-Control: Evidence from the Health Club Industry,"* mimeo, University of California, Berkeley.

Finkelstein, Daniel, Elaine Hill, & Robert Whitaker. (2008). "School Food Environments and Policies in U.S. Public Schools," *Pediatrics, 122(1)*, e25 1-e259.

Gordon, Anne, Mary Kay Fox, Melissa Clark, Renee Nogales, Elizabeth Condon, Philip Gleason, Ankur Sarin. (2007). *School Nutrition Dietary Assessment-III: Vol. II: Student Participation and Dietary Intakes*, prepared for U.S. Department of Agriculture, Food and Nutrition Service,

Office of Research, Nutrition, and Analysis, Project Officer: Patricia McKinney, November.

Just, David, Lisa Mancino, and Brian Wansink. (2007). *Could Behavioral Economics Help Improve Diet Quality for Nutrition Assistance Program Participants?* Economic Research Report No. 43, U.S. Department of Agriculture, Economic Research Service, June.

Laibson, David. (2004). "Golden Eggs and Hyperbolic Discounting," in *Advances in Behavioral Economics*, Colin F. Camerer, George Loewenstein, and Matthew Rabin (eds.), Russell Sage Foundation, Princeton, NJ: Princeton University Press, pp. 429-57.

Lin, Biing-Hwan, Joanne Guthrie, and Elizabeth Frazao. (2001). "American Children's Diets Not Making the Grade," *FoodReview, 24(2)*, 8-17, U.S. Department of Agriculture, Economic Research Service.

Loewenstein, George. (2004)."Out of Control: Visceral Influences on Behavior," in *Advances in Behavioral Economics,* Colin F. Camerer, George Loewenstein, and Matthew Rabin (eds.), Russell Sage Foundation, Princeton, NJ: Princeton University Press, 689-724.

Oliveira, Victor. (2006). *The Food Assistance Landscape: FY 2006 Midyear Report*, Economic Information Bulletin No. 6-3, U.S. Department of Agriculture, Economic Research Service, September.

O'Toole, Terrance P., Susan Anderson, Clare Miller, and Joanne Guthrie. (2007). "Nutrition Services and Foods and Beverages Available at School: Results from the School Health Policies and Programs Study 2006," *Journal of School Health* 77(8): 500-21.

Polivy, J., Herman, C. P., Hackett, R. & Kuleshnyk, I. (1986). "The Effects of Self-Attention and Public Attention on Eating in Restrained and Unrestrained Subjects," *Journal of Personality and Social Psychology, 50(6)*, 1253-60.

Ralston, Katherine, Constance Newman, Annette Clauson, Joanne Guthrie, and Jean Buzby. (2007). *The National School Lunch Program: Background, Trends, and Issues*, Economic Research Report No. 61, U.S. Department of Agriculture, Economic Research Service, July.

Shefrin, Hersh, M., & Richard, H. Thaler. (2004). "Mental Accounting, Saving and Self Control," in *Advances in Behavioral Economics,* Colin F. Camerer, George Loewenstein, and Matthew Rabin (eds.), Russell Sage Foundation, Princeton, NJ: Princeton University Press, 395-428.

Shiv, B. & Fedorikhin, A. (1999). "Heart and Mind in Conflict: Interplay of Affect and Cognition in Consumer Decision Making," *Journal of Consumer Research, 26(3)*, 278-92.

Story, Mary, Karen M. Kaphingst, and Simone French. (2006). "The Role of Schools in Obesity Prevention," *The Future of Children, 16(1)*, 109-42, accessed at http://www.futureof children.

Sunstein, Cass, & Richard Thaler. (2003). "Libertarian Paternalism Is Not an Oxymoron," *University of Chicago Law Review, 70(4)*, 1159-202.

Thaler, Richard H. (1980). "Towards a Positive Theory of Consumer Choice." *Journal of Economic Behavior and Organization, 1*, 39-60.

Thaler, Richard, H. (2004). "Mental Accounting Matters," in *Advances in Behavioral Economics,* Colin F. Camerer, George Loewenstein, and Matthew Rabin (eds.), Russell Sage Foundation, Princeton, NJ: Princeton University Press, 74-103.

Thaler, Richard, H. & Shlomo Benartzi. (2004). "Save More Tomorrow (TM): Using Behavioral Economics To Increase Employee Saving," *Journal of Political Economy, 112(S1)*, S 164-S 187, University of Chicago Press, February.

U.S. Department of Agriculture, Food and Nutrition Service. 2007. USDA Web site accessed at *http://www.fns.usda.gov/ fsp/rules*. htm on January 10, 2007.

Wansink, B. (2006). *Mindless Eating: Why We Eat More Than We Think,* New York: Bantam Dell.

CHAPTER SOURCES

The following chapters have been previously published:

Chapter 1 – This is an edited, excerpted and augmented edition of a University of Michigan study Contractor and Cooperator Report Number 54, dated July 2009.

Chapter 2 – This is an edited, excerpted and augmented edition of a supplement to a University of Michigan study Contractor and Cooperator Report Number 54, dated July 2009.

Chapter 3 – This is an edited, excerpted and augmented edition of a United States Department of Agriculture publication, Report Number 87, dated November 2009.

Chapter 4 – This is an edited, excerpted and augmented edition of a United States Department of Agriculture publication, Report Number 68, dated December 2008.

INDEX